HORIZONS IN CANCER RESEARCH

VOLUME 55

HORIZONS IN CANCER RESEARCH

Additional books in this series can be found on Nova's website
under the Series tab.

Additional e-books in this series can be found on Nova's website
under the e-book tab.

HORIZONS IN CANCER RESEARCH

VOLUME 55

HIROTO S. WATANABE
EDITOR

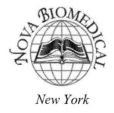

New York

Library of Congress Cataloging-in-Publication Data

ISSN: 2159-1326

ISBN: 978-1-63463-228-7

Published by Nova Science Publishers, Inc. † *New York*

Contents

Preface   **vii**

Chapter 1   Curcumin: A Folklore Remedy from Kitchen on the
                 Way to Clinic As Cancer Drug   **1**
                 Debasish Bandyopadhyay

Chapter 2   Diagnosis of Thyroid Cancers in the Era of Molecular
                 Medicine: New Paradigm in Cytologic and Histologic Diagnosis
                 of Thyroid Cancer?   **43**
                 Lewis A. Hassell, Ericka Olgaard and S. Terence Dunn

Chapter 3   The Potential Role of Arsenic Trioxide in the Treatment
                 of Iodine Non-Avid Thyroid Cancer   **71**
                 Eleonore Fröhlich and Richard Wahl

Chapter 4   Xerostomia: Causes, Prevention and Management   **101**
                 Hong Wu, M.D., M.S., Jennifer Yacub Martin, M.D.
                 and Dian Wang, M.D., Ph.D.

Chapter 5   Causes of Xerostomia in the Cancer Treatment   **123**
                 Eliana Aparecida Minicucci,
                 Silke Anna Theresa Weber
                 and Glenda Nicioli da Silva

Chapter 6   Psychoeducation: An Alternative for Preparing the
                 Cancer Patient's Primary Caregiver   **135**
                 Vivian Guerra Morales, Lisandra Angulo Gallo,
                 Zeida Castillo Díaz, Aguedo M. Treto González,
                 Maria Domingas Cassinda Vissupe,
                 Mayté González García, Rachel Fernández Ramos,
                 Ladisbel López Lorenzo and Patricia Gil Pérez

Index   **149**

Preface

This book presents original results on the leading edge of cancer research. Topics discussed include curcumin; diagnosis of thyroid cancers in the era of molecular medicine; xerostomia; the potential role of arsenic trioxide in the treatment of iodine non-avid thyroid cancer; causes of xerostomia in the cancer treatment; and an alternative for preparing the cancer patient's primary caregiver.

Chapter 1 – Numerous compounds are widely distributed in nature and many of these possess medicinal/biological/pharmacological activity. Curcumin, a polyphenol derived from the rhizomes (underground stems) of *Curcuma longa* Linn (a member of the ginger family, commonly known as turmeric) is a culinary spice and therapeutic used in India for thousands of years to induce color and flavor in food as well as to treat a wide array of diseases. The origin of turmeric as spice and folklore medicine is so old that it is lost in legend. Curcumin has many beneficial pharmacological effects which includes, but are not limited with, antimicrobial, anti-inflammatory, antioxidant, antiviral, antiangiogenic, and antidiabetic activities. Most importantly curcumin possesses immense antitumorigenic effect. It prevents tumor formation in a number of animal models, including models of lung, liver, stomach, colon, breast, esophageal cancer etc. A concise discussion regarding the effects of curcumin on five leading cancers with respect to cancer mortality (lung, liver, stomach, colorectal and breast) and associated molecular mechanisms is included. The potential applications of curcumin as chemopreventive agent, chemosensitizer, and radiosensitizer in both *in vitro* and *in vivo* studies have discussed in this chapter. In addition to natural drugs, a large number of synthetic drugs (mainly organic and organometallic) are being used as medicines against cancer. Synergistic role of two or more drugs against any particular disease plays an important role in modern drug discovery research. Subsequently, preclinical and clinical studies of drug synergy have become an intriguing part of translational research.

This chapter describes the pertinent recent examples of synergistic role of curcumin with various other molecules with special emphasis to commercial drugs and natural products. Curcumin has also demonstrated the ability to improve patient outcomes in clinical trials.

Chapter 2 – *Background:* The Bethesda system for standardized reporting of thyroid fine needle aspiration (FNA) cytology has positively impacted clarity of communication of results and management of patients evaluated for thyroid nodules. Problematic areas still exist in the triage of some of these samples, particularly those in the categories of "follicular lesion with atypia of uncertain significance" and "follicular lesion". The discovery of a variety of molecular markers associated with various thyroid neoplasms offers both opportunity and challenges in appropriate application to the patient with a thyroid nodule. Additionally, a transition from molecular marker to therapeutic target begins to change the treatment paradigm both before and following surgical intervention. *Methods:* The literature on molecular and genetic abnormalities in thyroid lesions is reviewed. Potentially useful markers for distinguishing currently problematic categories of FNA cytologic samples, especially non-diagnostic samples, atypia of uncertain significance, and follicular lesions are discussed. The predictive value of molecular analyses in these settings is examined. The role of molecular evaluation of resected tumors is also reviewed. *Results:* Evaluation of FNA samples with negative or suboptimal follicular cytology for Ras gene mutations may be useful in detecting potentially significant follicular lesions (carcinomas) but is quite low in overall yield. Cytologic samples with atypia of uncertain significance, as well as those classified as follicular lesions or suspicious for malignancy, which may include the possibility of papillary carcinomas, may be fruitfully evaluated using a panel of molecular tests for *BRAF, RET/*PTC, *PAX8/PPARγ1* and Ras genes. Other emerging markers have potential utility in the work-up of thyroid lesions.

Chapter 3 – Arsenic trioxide (ATO) is an approved second-line medication for acute promyelocytic leukemia (APL). A positive role for this drug in the treatment of solid carcinomas has been proposed but not established yet. According to clinical trials, solid cancers that might benefit from ATO treatment include melanoma, hepatocellular carcinoma, kidney, and hormone-refractory prostate cancers. In combination with other drugs positive effects have been reported for colorectal cancer. Animal models indicated efficacy in glioma or lung cancer and clinical trials have been performed. For thyroid cancer, anti-proliferative, proapoptotic and differentiating effects have been reported. Toxicity limits the use of ATO as a chemotherapeutic compound. Acute toxic effects during chemotherapy of APL have been described. Another issue in using ATO is its carcinogenicity. As the same mechanisms are involved both in the carcinogenic and therapeutic effects of ATO, it is mainly the dose applied and the cell type exposed to ATO that determines which cellular effect predominates. For the therapeutic efficacy of ATO, the most relevant effects are cell cycle arrest, induction of apoptosis through the mitochondrial pathway and autophagy. Additional anti-tumor effects include decreased tumor cell migration and invasion. ATO effects are mediated by activation of P3IK/Akt, MAP kinase and NfκB. Differentiating effects caused by ATO include suppression of tumor-relevant proteins such as cell cycle inhibitors, survivin, CD133, metalloproteinases, and upregulation of factors commonly suppressed in tumor cells, such as p53 and Fas. In addition, ATO also induces changes in cellular behaviour, such as decreased tumor cell invasion and increased iodide uptake in thyroid cancer. In the latter, radioiodine treatment of differentiated thyroid cancer is the preferred option after surgery to eliminate residual tumor cells. It is an efficient and selective treatment provided the neoplastic thyrocytes can accumulate iodide. Mutations and over-activity of PI3K/Akt and MAP kinase signalling is crucial in the development and progression of thyroid cancer and serve as targets for differentiating therapy. Differentiation therapy in thyroid cancer aims to restore iodide uptake and thereby increase sensitivity to radioiodine therapy. To achieve this goal a variety of compounds, such as retinoids, inhibitors of tyrosine kinases, of peroxisome proliferator-γ, of DNA methyltransferases, and of histone deacetylases are currently being evaluated in clinical trials. None of these single target inhibitors have produced optimal results. It is expected that multi-target compounds and combinations of substances will improve prognosis.

This review introduces arsenic as a toxic and therapeutic agent and illustrates its intracellular metabolism and its cellular targets for its carcinogenic and therapeutic effects. Results of ATO monotherapy and in combination with other compounds in solid cancer cell lines, in tumor xenografts and in clinical trials are reviewed. Based on the existing data, it can be concluded that monotherapy with ATO may not be promising for the treatment of solid cancers but combinations with other therapeutic interventions like ionizing radiation and thermo-therapy with iron oxide nanoparticles and synergism with cytostatic drugs might represent promising treatment options. In view of the specific relationship between the thyroid gland and arsenic, ATO might be a useful agent in the treatment of thyroid cancer.

Chapter 4 – Xerostomia, the subjective perception of dry mouth, is due to a variety of etiologies including polypharmacy, chemoradiation of head and neck cancers, systemic diseases and autoimmune disorders. It is associated with impaired swallowing, speech, taste, oral health, sleep and nutrition and thus can have a significant impact on a patient's quality of life. Given the significant effects of xerostomia, prevention and management of this symptom are of great importance in clinical practice. Prevention strategies are aimed at reducing the severity of xerostomia and are thus focused on reduction of radiation exposure, cytoprotectants, secretagogues and submandibular gland transfers. Treatment of xerostomia is challenging and unfortunately is not curative. Options for treatment include pharmacological agents, salivary substitutes, acupuncture, hyperbaric oxygen therapy, stimulants, oral care, and treatment of the underlying systemic or autoimmune disorder. Future investigations include gene transfer/therapy and stem cell replacement. The purpose of this chapter is to outline the causes, prevention and evidence based management of xerostomia to guide this undertreated clinical condition.

Chapter 5 – Saliva is fundamental for the maintenance of oral health. It is a complex mix of fluids secreted by major and minor salivary glands. Xerostomia is the subjective sensation of dry mouth, that can be associated or not to the diminution of the salivary flow. It predominantly affects middle aged and elderly people with an estimated prevalence of 21% and 27% in men and women, respectively. Oral dryness can profoundly affect the quality of life, interfering to basic daily functions such as chewing, swallowing and speaking. Reduction of volume and the antibacterial properties of saliva may cause infections, accelerate tooth decay and periodontal disease. The most important causes of xerostomia include factors that act on the salivary center in the central nervous system related to emotions; the autonomic nervous system caused by encephalitis, cerebral tumors, cerebral vascular accidents, neurosurgery or drugs; autoimmune disease, viral or bacteria salivary gland infections, radiotherapy and chemotherapy and the hydro–electrolytic balance related to cystic fibrosis, primary cirrhoses, sarcoidosis, amyloidosis, hypothireoidism and hemochromatosis. The oral epithelium has a high "turn over", therefore is one of the main places in which manifest the side effects of chemotherapy (CT) and head and neck radiotherapy (RT). The xerostomia caused by RT can be due to indirect damage to epithelial and connective tissue elements of the gland, or direct damage to salivary acini and ducts. High-dose chemotherapy may affect the salivary flow, principally in hematopoietic cell transplantation, total body irradiation and concurrent medications.

Chapter 6 – *Introduction:* Cancer is a chronic disease with a huge bio-psycho-social and spiritual impact not only for the patient but also for the caregiver, who generally does not have the preparation to deal with this difficult task. Objective: To evaluate the effectiveness of the psychoeducational guides (PG) for the preparation of the primary caregiver of children and adults with cancer. *Methods and procedures*: A pre-experimental, cross-sectional design, pre and post-test, was performed. The sample was selected intentionally and was formed by 95 caregivers, 42 children and 53 adults with oncological disease from different centers from the provinces of Havana, Villa Clara, Cienfuegos, Camaguey and Santiago de Cuba. For the study, methods such as observation, questionnaire and the psychological interview followed by a Likert scale were applied. For processing data, the Wilcoxon test, the qualitative analysis of verbalizations and the methodological triangulation were utilized. *Results:* The results showed differences between the variables before and after the implementation of the PG. After the implementation of the PG results show positive influence in the knowledge of the disease, coping styles and motivation for the role ($p < 0.05$) of caregivers. There were no changes in the adoption of positive ways of life ($p = 0.655$, $p > 0.05$) *Conclusion:* PG was effective in developing better care skills in primary caregivers of children and adults with cancer, regardless of their inclusion in psychosocial intervention programs.

In: Horizons in Cancer Research. Volume 55
Editor: Hiroto S. Watanabe

ISBN: 978-1-63463-228-7
© 2015 Nova Science Publishers, Inc.

Chapter 1

Curcumin: A Folklore Remedy from Kitchen on the Way to Clinic As Cancer Drug

*Debasish Bandyopadhyay**

Department of Chemistry, The University of Texas-Pan American,
Edinburg, Texas, US

Dedicated to Professor (Dr.) John Miller Trant

Abstract

Numerous compounds are widely distributed in nature and many of these possess medicinal/biological/pharmacological activity. Curcumin, a polyphenol derived from the rhizomes (underground stems) of *Curcuma longa* Linn (a member of the ginger family, commonly known as turmeric) is a culinary spice and therapeutic used in India for thousands of years to induce color and flavor in food as well as to treat a wide array of diseases. The origin of turmeric as spice and folklore medicine is so old that it is lost in legend. Curcumin has many beneficial pharmacological effects which includes, but are not limited with, antimicrobial, anti-inflammatory, antioxidant, antiviral, antiangiogenic, and antidiabetic activities. Most importantly curcumin possesses immense antitumorigenic effect. It prevents tumor formation in a number of animal models, including models of lung, liver, stomach, colon, breast, esophageal cancer etc. A concise discussion regarding the effects of curcumin on five leading cancers with respect to cancer mortality (lung, liver, stomach, colorectal and breast) and associated molecular mechanisms is included. The potential applications of curcumin as chemopreventive agent, chemosensitizer, and radiosensitizer in both *in vitro* and *in vivo* studies have

---

* Corresponding author: Debasish Bandyopadhyay. Department of Chemistry, The University of Texas-Pan American, 1201 West University Drive, Edinburg, Texas 78539, USA. Phone: +1(956)5789414, fax: +1(956) 3845006, e-mail: bandyopad@utpa.edu or dbomchem@gmail.com.

discussed in this chapter. In addition to natural drugs, a large number of synthetic drugs (mainly organic and organometallic) are being used as medicines against cancer. Synergistic role of two or more drugs against any particular disease plays an important role in modern drug discovery research. Subsequently, preclinical and clinical studies of drug synergy have become an intriguing part of translational research.

This chapter describes the pertinent recent examples of synergistic role of curcumin with various other molecules with special emphasis to commercial drugs and natural products. Curcumin has also demonstrated the ability to improve patient outcomes in clinical trials.

Keywords: Cancer, Carcinoma, Adenocarcinoma, Sarcoma, Neoplasm, Apoptosis, Angiogenesis, Cell death, Tumor, Toxicity, Carcinogenesis, Drug synergy, Synergistic effect, Natural products, Heterocycles, Medicinal chemistry, Pharmacophore, Pharmacology, Bioactive, Organometallics, Pharmaceutical

Abbreviations

3'-UTR	Three prime untranslated region
8-OHdG	8-Hydroxy-2'-deoxyguanosine
ACEI	Angiotensin converting enzyme inhibitor
AFM	Atomic force microscopy
AIN	American Institute of Nutrition
ALDH	Aldehyde dehydrogenase
AMP	Adenosine 5'-monophosphate
AMPK	Adenosine 5'-monophosphate (AMP)-activated protein kinase
Apaf-1	Apoptosis protease-activating factor-1
ARNT	Aryl hydrocarbon receptor nuclear translocator
ATG5	Autophagy protein 5
Bak	Bcl-2-antagonist/killer
Bax	B-cell lymphoma-2-associated X protein
Bcl- X_L	B-cell lymphoma-extra large
Bcl-2	B-cell lymphoma-2
Bcl-Xs	B-cell lymphoma-extra small
BRCA1	Breast cancer 1, early onset
CAF	Cancer-associated fibroblasts
CDK	Cyclin-dependent kinase
Chk1	Checkpoint kinase 1
CHOP	CCAAT/enhancer binding protein homologous protein
COX-2	Cyclooxygenase-2
CTNND1	Catenin delta-1
CTTN	Cortactin
CXCL1	Chemokine (C-X-C motif) ligand 1
DCLK1	Doublecortin-like kinase 1
DEN	Diethylnitrosamine

DIABLO	Direct inhibitor of apoptosis protein-binding protein with low isoelectric point
EGCG	(-)-Epigallocatechin-3-gallate
EGFR	Epidermal growth factor receptor
Egr-1	Early growth response-1
ER	Endoplasmic reticulum
ErbB-2	Erythroblastic leukemia viral oncogene homolog 2
Erk1/2	Extracellular signal-regulated kinase ½
EZH2	Enhancer of zeste homolog 2
FACS	Fluorescent activated cell sorter
FAS	Fatty acid synthase
FDA	Food and Drug administration (United States)
FOXO1	Forkhead box protein O1
GGTP	γ-Glutamyltranspeptidase
GSK3β	Glycogen synthase kinase 3β
HER2	Human epidermal growth factor receptor 2
HIF-1	Hypoxia-inducible factor-1
IGF-1R	Insulin-like growth factor 1 receptor
IL-8	Interleukin-8
IκBα	Inhibitor of nuclear factor of kappa light polypeptide gene enhancer in B-cells-α
JMJD2A	Jumoji domain containing 2A
JNK	c-Jun N-terminal kinase
KDM4C	Lysine (K)-specific demethylase 4C
MAPK	Mitogen-activated protein kinase
Maspin	Mammary serine protease inhibitor
MDR	Multidrug resistance
MEF	Mouse embryonic fibroblast
MMP	Matrix metalloproteinase
MMR	Mismatch repair
mRNA	Messenger RNA
MRP-1	Multidrug resistance-associated protein-1
MTT	3-[4,5-Dimethyl-2-thiazolyl]-2,5 diphenyltetrazolium bromide
NAFLD	Non-alcoholic fatty liver disease
NAT	*N*-acetyltransferase
NF-κB	Nuclear factor-κB
NSCLC	Non-small cell lung cancer
NTR	Neurotensin receptor
PAK1	Serine/threonine *p21-activated kinase 1*
PARP	Poly ADP ribose polymerase
p-EGFR	Phosphorylated epidermal growth factor receptor
p-Erk1/2	phosphorylated Extracellular signal related kinase ½
P-gp	P-glycoprotein
PKB	Protein kinase B (also known as Akt)
PP2A	Phosphatases 2A
PP5	Phosphatases 5

PPARα	Peroxisome proliferator-activated receptor-α
PRP4B	Pre-mRNA processing factor 4B
PTPN1	Protein tyrosine phosphatase, non-receptor type 1
Rac1	Ras-related C3 botulinum toxin substrate 1
RNAi	RNA interference
ROS	Reactive oxygen species
RT-PCR	Reverse transcription polymerase chain reaction
SCLC	Small cell lung cancer
siRNA	small interfering RNA
Smac	Second mitochondria-derived activator of caspase
SREBP-1c	Sterol regulatory element binding proteins-1c
STAT3	Signal transducer and activator of transcription 3
T790M	T790M mutation results in an amino acid substitution at position 790 in EGFR, from a threonine (T) to a methionine (M)
TGF β1	Transforming growth factor β1
TLR-4	Toll-like receptor-4
TNBC	Triple-negative breast cancer
TNF-α	Tumor necrosis factor-α
TOP2A	DNAtopoisomerase II alpha
TPA	12-O-tetradecanoylphorbol-13-acetate
VEGF	Vascular endothelial growth factor
VM	Vasculogenic mimicry
WHO	World Health Organization
α-SMA	α-Smooth muscle actin

1. Introduction

Natural products are intimate part of human civilization. It is impossible to say exactly when menfolk started to take plant portions to cure various diseases. Medicinal plants have been employed for thousands of years as remedies for human ailments because of the presence of particular phytochemicals. Phytochemicals are the broad spectrum of compounds derived from plants ("phyto" means plant in Greek). In practice, the term "phytochemicals" refers to a wide variety of compounds found in plants, but is mainly used to describe those plant natural products that may affect human/animal health, either in positive (as medicine) or negative (as narcotic/poison) manner. One of the important classes of phytochemicals consists of nutraceuticals. The term "nutraceutical" was formed by the portmanteau of two different words: nutrition and pharmaceutical. DeFelice (1989) defined [1] nutraceutical as "any substance that is a food or a parts of food, that provides medical or health benefits, including the prevention and treatment of disease". Later, the definition was modified by Health Canada and accordingly [2] nutraceutical is "a product isolated or purified from foods that is generally sold in medicinal forms not usually associated with food. A nutraceutical is demonstrated to have a physiological benefit or provide protection against chronic disease".

Polyphenols are a fundamental class of nutraceuticals which are widely used as chemotherapeutic, chemoprotective as well as chemopreventive agents. Polyphenols are important constituents of many fruits, vegetables and cooking spices.

Beverages like coffee, green and black tea, red wine, chocolate, nuts etcetera are good source of polyphenols. It has been found that many polyphenols are strong antioxidant, anti-inflammatory, cardioprotective, hepatoprotective and neuroprotective agents as well as immune regulators, either by itself on in combination with others [3]. Curcuminoids are a key category of polyphenols.

2. Origin and Historical Background

Curcumin (diferuloylmethane), the major constituent of curcuminoids, is present in turmeric which is the dried powered rhizomes (underground stems) of *Curcuma longa* Linn of the Zingiberaceae family. The medicinal use of turmeric (haridra) was indicated in Sushruta Samhita, one of the three fundamental texts of Ayurveda (Indian traditional medicine) in the 6th century BCE. Its medicinal uses were also found in Charaka Samhita (300-500 BCE). As Indian traditional medicine (Ayurveda) turmeric has been using to treat a broad range of common disorders for over 6000 years [4].

In India, turmeric is used as a cooking spice to induce nice yellow-orange color and flavor in curries, pickles and chutneys. It is used worldwide as a color inducing agent as well as preservative in American mustard, mayonnaise, butter and margarine and has been designated as international food additive E100 [5]. Turmeric is in the GRAS (Generally Recognized As Safe) list of the US Food and Drug Administration having GRN number 460 [6]. This royal spice was introduced to the western world in the 13th century by Marco Polo, one of the early European explorers to the Indian subcontinent [7, 10]. Since then India is the highest turmeric producing country in the world [8-10]. Turmeric has at least 76 synonyms listed in the 1999 World Health Organization (WHO) monograph [11]. A few popular names are Haridra (Sanskrit), Halood (Bengali), Haldi (Hindi), Kurkum uqdah safra (Arabic), Ukon (Japanese), Chiang Huang (Chinese), Ulgeum (Korean), Kurkuma (German), Safran des Indes (French), kurkumy (Russian), Indian saffron etc.

Besides its culinary appeal turmeric has a glorious history of uses as a therapeutic and preventive agent against a wide array of disorders and diseases, either by itself or in combination with other agents. As an ancient household remedy a hot poultice of turmeric powder and slaked lime (*chun-halood* in Bengali) is applied locally to relieve muscular pain and inflammation caused by sprain and injury.

In some parts of India, a drink made from fresh turmeric, ginger roots and honey in a glass of hot milk are given to women twice daily after childbirth.

A poultice of fresh turmeric paste is also applied to the perineum as wound healing for lacerations in the birth canal [12]. Its traditional uses as strong therapeutic or preventive agent against several human diseases include, but are not limited to, diabetes, fibrosis, asthma, rheumatism, allergies, inflammation, intestinal worms, atherosclerosis, diarrhea, dyspepsia, intermittent fevers, biliousness, cough, sinusitis, constipation, jaundice, urinary discharges, flatulence, leukoderma, amenorrhoea, acne, colic inflammation, respiratory ailments, lupus nephritis, irritable bowel syndrome, menstrual difficulties, anorexia, coryza, hematuria, hemorrhage, neurodegenerative, Alzheimer's disease, and cancer [9, 12-16]. The presence of turmeric is essential in most of the religious ceremonies in Hinduism.

The sequence of curcumin in natural product chemistry can be accessed as:

Natural products → Plant natural products → Phytochemicals → Nutraceuticals → Polyphenols → Curcuminoids → Curcumin

In the same way the categorization of *Curcuma longa* Linn is shown in Table 1.

Depending upon the soil composition and geographical diversity, the chemical composition of turmeric varies to some extent.

Table 1. Classification of *Curcuma longa*

Kingdom:	Plantae
Division:	Magnoliophyta
Class:	Liliopsida
Subclass:	Zingiberidae
Order:	Zingiberales
Family:	Zingiberaceae
Genus:	*Curcuma*
Species:	*C. longa*
Scientific Name:	*Curcuma longa*

The presence of about 235 compounds of which 109 sesquiterpenes, 68 monoterpenes, 22 diarylheptanoids and diarylpentanoids, 8 phenylpropene and other phenolic compounds, 5 diterpenes, 4 sterols, 3 triterpenoids, 2 alkaloids and 14 other compounds have been identified in turmeric. Among the diarylheptanoids three compounds are curcuminoids, the major pharmacologically active ingredients of turmeric. Curcumin, the major curcuminoid which constitutes 3-5% of turmeric has been consumed for medicinal purposes for thousands of years [14, 17]. Two other curcuminoids are demethoxycurcumin and *bis*-demethoxycurcumin (Figure 1). Commercial curcumin is a mixture of three curcuminoids: curcumin (71.5%), demethoxycurcumin (19.4%) and *bis*-demethoxycurcumin (9.1%) [14].

The isolation of curcumin, the principal constituent of turmeric responsible for its vibrant yellow-orange color, first reported by Vogel and Pelletier [18] in 1815 from the plant *Curcuma longa* as "yellow coloring-matter" and named as "curcumin". Later, it was found to be a mixture of resin and turmeric oil [19]. Curcumin was isolated in 1842 but the chemical formula was not reported [19, 20]. The chemical structure of curcumin as diferuloylmethane was identified by Milobedzka et al. in 1910 and the first synthesis of curcumin was reported from the same laboratory in 1913 [19, 21, 22]. The chemical structure of curcumin was confirmed in 1973 [23] and a few years ago in 2007, its solution structure was reported [24].

There are at least 125 plants under the genus *Curcuma* but curcuminoids have been identified only from 7 *Curcuma* plants [3, 10, 25, 26] till date.

As mentioned earlier, *Curcuma longa* Linn is the major source (3-5% curcuminoids) of curcuminoids and curcumin. Curcuminoids are also reported from *C. phaeocaulis* (1-3% curcuminoids), *C. xanthorrhiza* (1-2% curcuminoids), *C. zedoaria* (~ 0.1% curcuminoids), *C.*

aromatic (< 0.1% curcuminoids), *C. comosa* (< 0.1% curcuminoids), and *C. mangga* (< 0.1% curcuminoids). Curcuminoids have also been identified in other genera like *Costus speciosus, Etlingera elatior, Zingiber cassumunar* etc.

Besides the ancient literature, the first scientific report related to the medicinal uses of *Curcuma* was published in 1748 [27, 28]. After 67 years a review detailing the biological and medicinal properties of turmeric (curcumin) was published [18]. In 1937, Oppenheimer reported the medicinal activity of turmeric against biliary diseases [29].

In 1949, Schraufstatter and Bernt reported [30] the antibacterial activity of curcumin and its pharmacological activity to cure eye disease was reported [31] by Chaudhri in the following year. Jiang and co-workers evaluated the anticancer activity of four natural products *viz.* camptothecin, harringtonin, cantharidin and curcumin on human tumor biopsies in an *in vitro* soft agar clonogenic assay system and reported their findings in 1983 [32].

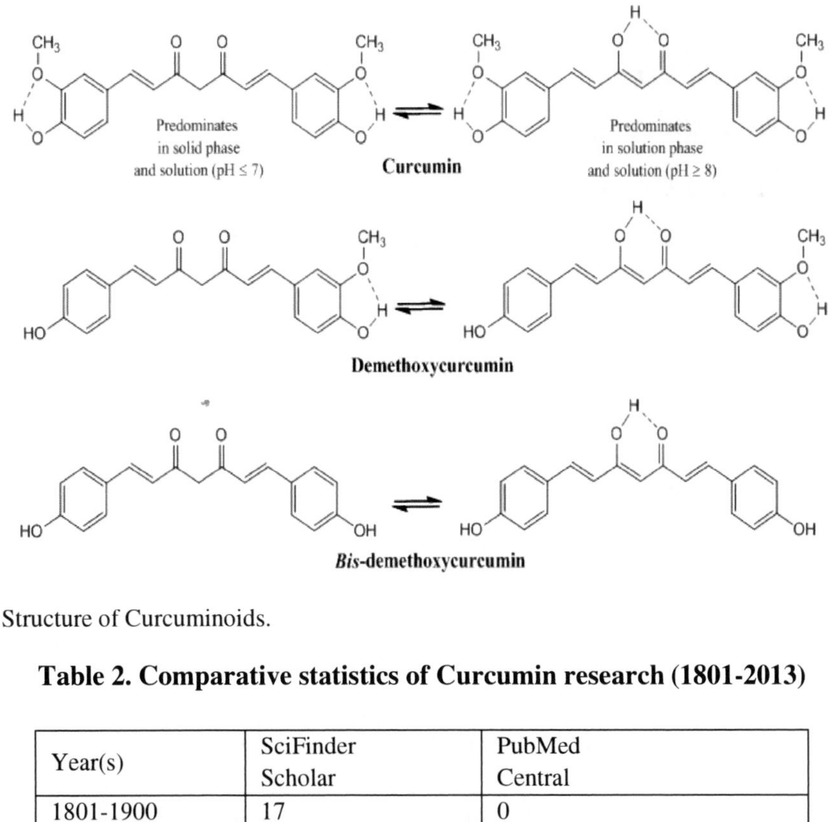

Figure 1. Structure of Curcuminoids.

Table 2. Comparative statistics of Curcumin research (1801-2013)

Year(s)	SciFinder Scholar	PubMed Central
1801-1900	17	0
1901-1950	92	1
1951-1980	373	6
1981-1990	264	5
1991-2000	1101	75
2001-2010	7073	2505
2011	1576	1282
2012	1948	1637
2013	1797	1233

[keyword: curcumin].

They reported curcumin as "relatively ineffective" antitumor agent than camptothecin, and harringtonin. Probably this was the first evaluation of curcumin against cancer. Kuttan and colleagues published the anticancer activity of curcumin in 1985 [33].

The acceptance of traditional medicine is considered as an alternative form of modern health care system. Over the past quarter century there has been growing interest in a possible role of curcumin on various diseases. The research topic "curcumin" in any chemistry/health related search engine hits a huge number of results, including research articles, reviews, communications, patents, books, editorials etc. Comparative results obtained up to December 31, 2013 from the two major chemistry and health related databases *viz.* SciFinder Scholar and PubMed Central are presented in Table 2 and Figure 2. After publication of the initial studies on curcumin as a promising anticancer agent in the mid-eighties [32, 33], scientists from all over the world paid their attention to this novel nutraceutical. It is now established that cancer is neither a single disease nor a comparatively new disease.

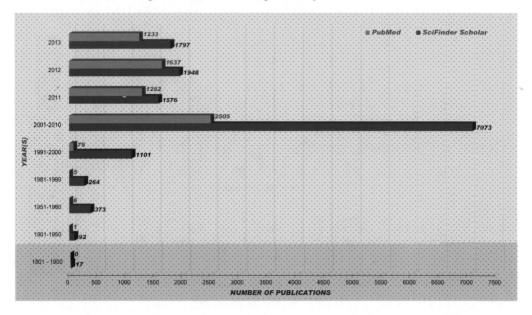

Figure 2. Growing interest (comparative statistics) on Curcumin research.

3. Curcumin and Cancer

It is well-known that cancer is a leading cause of death worldwide and accounted for 8.2 million deaths in 2012 among which 70% occur in low and middle income countries. According to the World Health Organization the annual cancer cases will rise from 14 million in 2012 to 22 within the next two decades [34, 35].

On the other hand, cancer is a group of more than 200 neoplastic diseases caused by the dysregulation of multiple factors [36]. Therefore, there is a continuous need to introduce new anticancer agents to reduce both cancer incidence and cancer-related mortalities.

Moreover, cancer cells often adapt to develop resistance to chemotherapeutic agents, consequently a better understanding of anticancer agents induce or inhibit carcinogenesis could lower tumor incidence or provide help to manage this disease effectively. Current research in this field directs to develop novel chemotherapeutic agents, which are more potent tumor-selective cytotoxic agents and can circumvent drug resistant cancer cells. A tentative estimation states that about 25% drugs are still derived from the Mother Nature and 74-80% of all cancer drugs have their origins in natural products i.e. these drugs are *modified natural products* [37, 38].

Several scientists around the world are actively engaged to investigate the anticancer activity of the ancient natural product curcumin. Consequently a huge number of publications detailing its anticancer activity have been published. A concise discussion regarding the effects of curcumin on five leading cancers with respect to cancer mortality *viz.* lung, liver, stomach, colorectal and breast (Figure 3) can be found in the sequel. The outcome of some important and comparatively recent studies have been summarized in this chapter.

3.1. Lung Cancer

The overall percentages of occupancy (13.0) and mortality (19.4) of lung cancer were highest worldwide among all cancers in 2012 [34, 35, 39]. About 85-90% lung cancers are non-small cell lung carcinoma (NSCLC) and 5-year prevalence is only 5.8%. The chemotherapeutic and chemopreventive activities of curcumin against lung cancer have been reported. Singh and co-workers reported [40] that Curcumin can behave as a potential adjuvant chemotherapeutic agent against NSCLC by enhancing chemotherapeutic effect of the drug Vinorelbine (trade name Navelbine) in H520 cells *in vitro*. Independent treatment of Cucumin and Vinorelbine induced 23.7% and 38% apoptosis respectively whereas pretreatment with Curcumin amplified Vinorelbine induced apoptosis to 61.3%.

The mechanism of action suggested that Curcumin triggered apoptosis by enhancing the protein expression of Bax and Bcl-Xs while the protein expression of Bcl-2 and Bcl-X_L was reduced. Consequently, release of apoptogenic Cytochrome c took place, and the activity of Caspase-9 and Caspase-3 boosted. Here it is important to mention that Bcl-X_L is a protein consisted by 233-amino acids associated with antiapoptotic properties.

On the other hand, one of the alternatively spliced transcripts of the B*cl-x* gene codes for the protein Bcl-x_S, which lacks 63 amino acids present in Bcl-x_L and associated with proapoptotic activity. Lev-Ari et al. exposed the non-small cell lung cancer PC-14 cells for 72h to curcumin (0-50 μM) and apoptosis was determined by FACS analysis. Finally, the COX-2, EGFR, ErbB-2 and p-Erk1/2 expressions were measured by Western blot analysis. The results showed that inhibitory effect of Curcumin on survival and apoptosis of lung cancer cell lines was significantly higher in the COX-2-expressing cells than in the COX-2-deficient cells. Curcumin decreased COX-2, EGFR and p-Erk1/2 expressions in a dose-dependent manner [41]. Radhakrishna-Pillai et al. demonstrated Curcumin-induced apoptosis in two human lung cancer cell lines A549 (adenocarcinomic human alveolar basal epithelial cells) and H-1299 (also known as NCI-H1299 or CRL-5803).

Upon Curcumin treatment the growth of both the cell lines was inhibited in time and concentration dependent manner [42]. In the presence of 40 mM curcumin a decrease in expression of p53, bcl-2, and bcl-X_L was observed after 12 h exposure while *Bak* and *Caspase* genes remained unchanged up to 60 mM curcumin but showed decrease in expression levels at 80 – 160 mM. It was suggested that the apoptotic cell death by curcumin involves multiple pathways. Curcumin up-regulates various pro-apoptotic genes and simultaneously down-regulate some of the anti-apoptotic genes. Homo-dimerization or hetero-dimerization of these pro- and anti-apoptotic genes in favor of apoptosis was one of the suggested mechanisms of Curcumin-induced apoptosis. The mechanistic pathway by which Bax and Bak, two multidomain pro-apoptotic Bcl-2 family members, regulate curcumin-induced apoptosis was revealed by Shankar et al. [43]. The study involved the use of mouse embryonic fibroblasts (MEFs) deficient in *Bax*, *Bak* or both genes. The treatment with Curcumin caused an escalation in the protein levels of both *Bax* and *Bak*, and mitochondrial translocation.

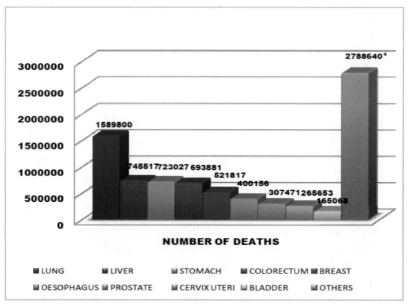

*All cancers excluding non-melanoma skin cancer. Specific type of cancer and its percentage of contribution toward cancer related mortality in 2012 can be shortened [39] as: Lip, oral cavity (1.8), Nasopharynx (0.6), Other pharynx (1.2), Gallbladder (1.7), Pancreas (4.1), Larynx (1.1), Melanoma of skin (0.7), Kaposi sarcoma (0.3), Corpus uteri (0.9), Ovary (1.9), Testis (0.1), Kidney (1.7), Brain, nervous system (2.3), Thyroid (0.5), Hodgkin lymphoma (0.3), Non-Hodgkin lymphoma (2.4), Multiple myeloma (1.0), Leukaemia (3.2).

Figure 3. Mortality due to Cancer in 2012 (worldwide).

Consequently mitochondrial membrane potential dropped which favored the cytosolic release of apoptogenic molecules such as Cytochrome c and Smac/DIABLO from mitochondria to cytosol to activate caspase-9 and caspase-3 and eventually apoptosis. The authors also suggested that Curcumin-induced caspase activation might be amplified due to induction of Apaf-1 because it also caused an increase in the protein level of Apaf-1 in wild-type MEFs. Taken together, both Bax and Bak are essential for curcumin-induced apoptosis, and over-expression of Smac/DIABLO as interventional approach to combat with Bax-and/or Bak-deficient chemoresistant cancers for curcumin-based therapy.

Cisplatin (or cisplatinum, or *cis*-diamminedichloroplatinum[II]) has been using as a novel anticancer drug against several types of cancer for the past more than three decades (Figure 4, Synthesis: 1970; FDA approval: 1978).

However, the efficiency of Cisplatin-based chemotherapy can't reach to its expected level; because of *de novo* drug resistance in the advanced stage of cancer or in cancer cells acquiring cisplatin resistance during therapy. It has been found that the late detection and growing drug resistance are the two main causes of high mortality due to lung cancer [39].

Under this circumstances, the chemosensitization strategy might be beneficial to fight against lung cancer. As an excellent chemosensitizer, Curcumin can sensitize Cisplatin-mediated apoptosis in human non-small cell lung cancer H460 cells.

The mechanism involves the generation of superoxide anion and down-regulation of the anti-apoptotic Bcl-2 protein through proteasomal degradation and subsequent sensitization of the cancer cells to Cisplatin-assisted apoptosis.

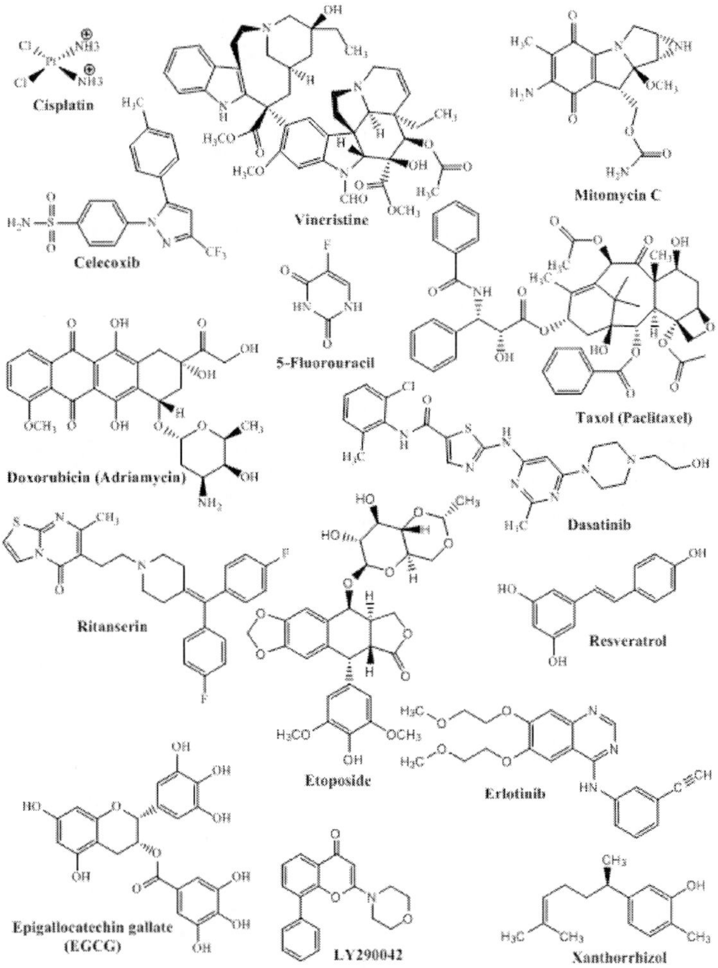

Figure 4. Example of drugs demonstrated synergistic effect with Curcumin.

In a nutshell, treatment of the non-small cell lung cancer H460 cells with Cisplatin using Curcumin as chemosensitizer resulted in reversal of Bcl-2-facilitated cisplatin resistance and consequently increased apoptosis [44].

Not only as chemotherapeutic and/or chemosensitizing agent, Curcumin also demonstrated its chemopreventive activity immensely against lung cancer. It is known that

TNF-α and oxidants activate transcription factors such as NF-κB, which is involved in the transcription of proinflammatory mediators, including Interleukin 8 (IL-8).

It was found [45] that the treatment of cultured alveolar epithelial cells (A549) with hydrogen peroxide (100 μM) and TNF-α (10 ng/ml) the NF-κB and activator protein-1 (AP-1) activation were increased significantly and IL-8 was released. The treatment with Curcumin inhibited both hydrogen peroxide and TNF-α-mediated activation of NF-κB and AP-1; the release of IL-8 was inhibited also.

Moreover, an increased level of glutathione and glutamylcysteine ligase catalytic subunit mRNA expression were observed in curcumin-treated A549 cells in comparison to untreated cells.

The study suggested that curcumin contains multiple properties like (i) it can act as an oxygen radical scavenger, (ii) antioxidant through modulation of glutathione levels, and (iii) anti-inflammatory agent through inhibition of IL-8 release in lung cells. It is known that the drug Erlotinib (an EGFR-tyrosine kinase inhibitor, Figure 4) can produce satisfactory result in human lung adenocarcinoma PC-9 cells by inducing apoptosis. However Erlotinib exhibited weaker effect on Erlotinib-resistant H1975 (or NCI-H1975) and H1650 (NCI-H1650) human lung cancer cells than Curcumin pretreated Cisplatin. The combination of Curcumin and Erlotinib showed similar effects on apoptosis as the combination of Curcumin and Cisplatin in Erlotinib-resistant non-small cell lung cancer cell lines. In addition, this combination (Curcumin and Erlotinib) significantly increased the cytotoxicity of Erlotinib to Erlotinib-resistant NSCLC cells and reduced the tumor growth in xenograft mouse model. The mechanism of action involves the down-regulation of the expressions of EGFR, p-EGFR, and survivin, and inhibition of the NF-κB activation by sustaining IκB expression level in Erlotinib-resistant NCI-H1650 and NCI-H1975 cells [46]. The primary reason of Erlotinib-resistance in lung cancer includes T790M mutant EGFR receptor and c-Met gene amplification. It has been found [47] that coadministration of Curcumin and Erlotinib in PC-9 lung cancer cells accelerated apoptosis by elevation of IκB expression. Also the coadministration of Curcumin and Erlotinib to siRNA-pretreated PC-9 lung cancer cells significantly increased the cytotoxicity by reducing the cell viability because of synergistic effect. This combination remarkably reduced the tumor growth in mice. The efficacy of Curcumin on the growth and metastasis of H1975 (NSCLC) in an intralung tumor mouse model has been reported [48] using ectopic and orthotopic lung tumor mouse models. The control group was given AIN-076 control diet whereas the investigating group received same food in addition to 0.6% curcumin 14 days prior to cell implantation and until the end of the experiment. The orthotopic tumor was generated by percutaneous injection of the lung cancer cells in Matrigel into the left lung of CD-1 nude mice. The successive Western blot analysis exhibited that the expressions of IkB, nuclear p65, COX-2 and p-ERK1/2 were down-regulated by curcumin *in vitro*. A 36% decrease in weight of intralung tumors of orthotopic human NSCLC xenografts with sufficient increase in survival rate of the investigating group was observed. Cigarette smoke is considered as one of the main reasons of lung carcinogenesis. The presence of carcinogens such as Benzo[a]pyrene, the free radicals like hydroxyl radicals, superoxide radicals have the required potential to activate NF-κB which can inhibit apoptosis, stimulate proliferation and mediate tumorigenesis. Accordingly NF-κB is an ideal target for preventing cigarette smoke-mediated lung carcinogenesis. The effect of Curcumin on cigarette smoke-induced NF-κB activation and NF-κB-regulated gene expression was studied in H1299 (human non-small cell lung carcinoma), A549 (human lung epithelial cell carcinoma), and BEAS-2B (immortalized human bronchial epithelial) cells [49]. The results showed that pre-treatment with curcumin stopped the cigarette smoke-prompted DNA-binding of NF-κB and NF-κB-dependent reporter gene expression.

Tissue invasion and metastasis are considered as one of the hallmarks in cancer. It has been found that relapse and/or metastasis are very common for lung cancer patients after complete excision of the cancer, even if they were at stage IA [50]. The protein Rac1 is widely related in cytoskeleton rearrangements (occur in physiological events such as cell movement. Cytoskeletal defects are frequently associated with cancer metastasis.) and migration, invasion as well as metastasis of cancer cells. Curcumin inhibits EGF or TGF β1-induced 801D lung cancer cell migration and invasion [51].

The decrease in the metastasis in curcumin-treated cells was anticipated due to the inhibition of Rac1/PAK1 pathway signaling and the decreased MMP-2 and MMP-9 expression. The anti-invasion activity of curcumin was confirmed by the relation between Rac1 and the growth and metastasis inhibitory effect of curcumin *in vivo* by the xenograft model. In another investigation [52] the growth inhibitory effect of Curcumin in both the non-small cell lung cancer (A549) and small cell lung cancer (SCLC) H460 (human) cell lines have been reported. The study suggested that Curcumin can prevent cell proliferation by the upregulation of CDK inhibitors, p27 and p21, and downregulation of Cyclin D1 although the compound precludes progression and metastasis through induction of FOXO1.

An interesting synergism of Curcumin with another important phytochemical Resveratrol (*trans*-3,5,4'-Trihydroxystilbene, Figure 4) against lung carcinogenesis has also been reported [53]. The Benzo[a]pyrene treatment in mice resulted in a substantial increase in the protein expression of phosphorylated p53 [specifically at ser15] which confirmed p53 hyper-phosphorylation while enzyme activities of caspase 3 and caspase 9 were observed to be potentially reduced. The combined treatment of Curcumin and Resveratrol to benzo[a]pyrene treated mice resulted in a significant decrease in p53 hyper-phosphorylation as well as regulation of cellular metabolism enzymes and caspases.

3.2. Liver Cancer

Liver cancer was the second leading cause of cancer related deaths (9.1%) worldwide in 2012 which accounted only 1.9% five-year prevalence [39]. In general, hepatocellular carcinoma is resistant to standard chemotherapy. Surgery or liver transplantation at the early stage may provide longer survival to the patients. However, about 80% of liver cancer patients with advanced stage are not amenable to liver transplantation or surgery and this is the main reason of poor prognosis in liver cancer [54]. Hence it is highly challenging to identify/develop effective drug to combat liver cancer. Curcumin demonstrated its antiproliferative activity against human HCC (hepatocellular carcinoma) cells by arresting the cell cycle in G2 and regulating Wnt signaling pathway [55]. The proliferation is inhibited by apoptosis in a dose-dependent manner. The interruption of Wnt signaling takes place by reduction of β-catenin activity, which in other word suppresses the expression of β-catenin target genes (*VEGF, Cyclin D1* and *c-myc*). The Wnt signaling pathway is considered as an important factor for the development, growth, survival, proliferation and metastasis of the cancer cells. The GSK3β and β-catenin play the major role in this pathway and therefore, a few factors associated with this pathway are considered as potential targets for anticancer therapy. Curcumin demonstrated the anti-migratory activity by suppressing the TPA-induced activation of the Wnt signaling and the related cell migration in Hep3B liver cancer cells [56] *in vitro* and tumor growth *in vivo*.

The molecular mechanism of Curcumin-induced apoptosis in human liver cancer (Huh7) cells was studied [57]. It is known that Fas ligand (FasL or CD95L) is a type-II transmembrane protein that belongs to TNF (tumor necrosis factor) family. Upon Curcumin treatment of Huh7 cells significant increase in Fas and FasL, caspase-3 activation as well as PARP cleavage have been observed. Rapid activation of p-38 under the influence of Curcumin triggers apoptosis *via* p-38-dependent up-regulation of FasL. High expression of FAS is associated with many types of cancer including liver cancer.

It has been found that Curcumin can down-regulate FAS expression to inhibit its intracellular activity and mRNA level in a concentration-dependent manner in HepG2 liver cancer cells *in vitro*. Curcumin induced apoptosis in HepG2 liver cancer cells with the IC_{50} value of 8.84 µg/mL determined by MTT assay. Not only FAS, the siRNA also showed similar result with Curcumin [58]. From flowcytometric analysis it was concluded that up-regulation of the expression of tubulin occurred by the treatment with Curcumin in HepG2 liver cancer cells. Treatment with Curcumin caused cell-cycle arrest at G2/M phase with concomitant losses from G0/G1 phase in a concentration-dependent manner.

The AFM imaging demonstrated that the membrane toxicity and cytoskeleton destruction may be the therapeutic targets of Curcumin [59].

It has been cited in many literatures that during oxidative stress the expression of TLR-4 is regulated. Excessive intracellular ROS production up-regulates TLR-4/2 expression whereas elimination of ROS by specific scavengers inhibits the up-regulation of TLR-4 expression and suppresses transcription of TLR-4 mediated genes. Therefore it is considered that ROS triggers the TLR-4 signaling pathway [60]. On the other hand, Myd-88 is a down-stream adaptor molecule of TLR-4 to conduct signals to begin translocation of NF-κB and activation of MAPKs which ultimately leads to cell death *via* apoptosis. The initiator of the caspase cascade, caspase-8, is activated by cleavage through the interaction with Fas-linked death domain *via* Myd-88. The executor of apoptosis in caspase cascade, caspase-3, can also be activated by cleavage after the activation of caspase-8 [61]. Curcumin-induced inhibition of cell proliferation as well as cell death through apoptosis in MHCC97H human liver cancer cell lines followed the sequence: activation of ROS $\rightarrow$ TLR4/Myd-88 $\rightarrow$ activation of Caspase-3/Caspase-8 [62]. The apoptosis occurred in a dose-dependent manner through activating intracellular ROS generation. The augmented intracellular ROS formation stimulated the TLR-4/MyD-88 signaling pathway.

Consequently the activation of caspase-8 and caspase-3 surfaced, which ultimately led to apoptosis in MHCC97H human liver cancer cells.

Vasculogenic mimicry (VM) is considered as one of the major factors in cancer invasion and it denotes the process in which the cancer cells mimic endothelial cells by forming blood channels. The potential of Curcumin on vasculogenic mimicry of human liver adenocarcinoma cells (SK-Hep-1) has been studied *in vitro*. Curcumin inhibited vasculogenic mimicry, decreased cell migration and MMP9 (matrix metalloproteinase-9) production of the cancer cells. Curcumin exhibited the anti-VM efficacy by down-regulating the Akt (or PKB) and STAT3 signaling pathways [63].

Two-dimensional electrophoresis and mass spectral investigations were carried out to reveal the effect of Curcumin on the proteome of human liver cancer HepG2 cell lines [64].

The HepG2 cells were treated with Curcumin (30 μmol/L) and the proteins were separated. An up-regulation of cyclin-dependent kinase inhibitor 2A, carnitine deficiency-associated gene, replication protein A2 and protein disulfide isomerase was noted whereas down-regulation of Nm23 protein, Stathmin 1/oncoprotein 18, Ran binding protein 1, endoplasmic reticulum-60 protease and proliferating cell nuclear antigen were noted. The data indicated that Curcumin treatment might led to inhibit tumor growth, promote apoptosis by arresting cell cycle, and prevent tumor invasion as well as metastasis.

The anti-atherosclerosis and hypolipidemic efficiencies of Curcumin might correlate with promotion of the transmembrane transport of fatty acids and maintain the stability of the cell membrane.

Hypoxia of solid tumor is one of the major problems to treat cancer. This situation arises when the cells are deprived of required oxygen. As a tumor develops, it promptly outgrows its blood supply, leaving portions of the tumor with areas where the oxygen concentration is significantly lower than in healthy tissues. Hypoxic microenvironements in solid tumors are in result of available oxygen being consumed within 70 to 150 μm of tumor vasculature by fast growing tumor cells thus limiting the amount of oxygen available to diffuse further into the tumor tissue. To support continuous growth and cell proliferation in hypoxic environments, cancer cells are found to alter their metabolism. Hypoxia-inducible factor-1 (HIF-1) plays a key role in cellular responses to hypoxia counting the transcriptional activation of a number of genes those are involved in tumor angiogenesis [65]. HIF-1 is composed of HIF-1a and aryl hydrocarbon receptor nuclear trans-locator (ARNT). It was reported that between these two subunits of HIF-1; ARNT was found to be attacked by curcumin in several cancer cell types, including mice bearing Hep3B liver cancer cell lines and in xenografted tumors. Curcumin activated the proteasomal degradation of ARNT through oxidation and ubiquitination processes to suppress ARNT, erythropoietin, and VEGF (a major HIF-1 target angiogenic factor) leading to overall down-regulation of HIF-1 in tumors [66]. In brief, the study showed that the anticancer effect of Curcumin in tumor hypoxia was because of ARNT degradation which caused HIF-1 inactivation. In the case of human liver cancer (HepG2) cells *in vitro* Curcumin treatment significantly reduced the hypoxia-mediated HIF-1 protein level by repressing the expression of VEGF in vascular endothelial cells which eventually inactivated the transcriptional activity of HIF-1 under hypoxia. Consequently, curcumin efficiently blocked the hypoxia-stimulated angiogenesis of vascular endothelial cells. These findings supported that Curcumin might play major roles in tumor suppression through the inhibition of HIF-1-mediated angiogenesis [66].

It has been stated earlier that the invasion of cancer cells is considered as an important and distinctive step toward metastasis. The blockage of this physiological incident by medicines or supplements/nutraceuticals prolongs the life span of an affected host. Kozuki et al. suggested [67] that antioxidative property of Curcumin might be involved in its anti-invasive effect. The authors evaluated the efficacy of Curcumin on the proliferation and invasion of the rat ascites hepatoma AH109A cells *in vitro* and *ex vivo*. To satisfy this goal, a co-culture system of the hepatoma cells with mesothelial cells derived from rat mesentery was subjected for invasion study. Curcumin reduced the hepatoma slipping motility in a concentration-dependent manner up to 5 μM and afterward maintained the effect up to 20 μM with a minimum impact on cell proliferation.

Interestingly, the sera isolated from rats, those consumed Curcumin orally, also inhibited the AH109A cellular invasion when added to the culture medium. Curcumin and curcumin-containing rat sera inhibited the ROS-potentiated invasive capacity by concurrently treating AH109A cells with hypoxanthine, xanthine oxidase and either of Curcumin samples.

Curcumin demonstrated synergism with other anticancer agents against a number of cancers including liver cancer. Curcumin along with EGCG (a natural polyphenol, mainly present in green tea, white tea and in black tea with low abundance, Figure 3) exhibited inhibition against acrylamide (a proven rodent carcinogen)-induced human liver cancer HepG2 cell proliferation. Acrylamide (≤ 100 μM) induced CYP2E1 expression potentially and knockdown of CYP2E1 restrained acrylamide to increase viability of HepG2 cells [68]. Moreover, acrylamide up-regulated EGFR, Cyclin D1 and NF-κB, which contributed to cell proliferation.

Curcumin and EGCG successfully down-regulated the protein expression of CYP2E1, EGFR, Cyclin D1 and NF-κB signaling pathway. Accordingly subsequent inhibition of acrylamide-induced HepG2 cell proliferation was observed. Prevention of angiogenesis signifies a fascinating approach to hepatocellular carcinoma as it is one of the hypervascular solid tumors. Curcumin demonstrated synergistic effect in combination with two other drugs namely: leflunomide (an antirheumatic drug) and perindopril, an angiotensin converting enzyme inhibitor (ACEI), against DEN-induced hepatocellular carcinoma in mice [69]. DEN was administered to the mice for a period of eight weeks and a notable increase in immunohistochemical staining of CD31-positive endothelial cells and consequently hepatic microvessel density (MVD) was observed as compared to normal liver. Following the trend, up-regulation of HIF-1α and VEGF was noticed in the DEN-treated mice in comparison to their normal counterpart. Monotherapy with leflunomide and perindopril showed week inhibition whereas Curcumin demonstrated down-regulation of HIF-1α.

The combined therapy of these three agents (Curcumin, leflunomide and perindopril) resulted synergism through suppression of VEGF expression and exhibiting inhibitory action on neovascularization and subsequent inhibition of angiogenesis. Nowadays it is well-known that metastasis of liver is a major cause of mortality in colorectal cancer (CRC). Curcumin in combination with ulinastatin (a glycoprotein which acts as urinary trypsin inhibitor) inhibited CRC liver metastases in human colorectal cancer cell lines HCT-116 *in vitro* through modulation of MMP-9 and expression of E-cadherin. Because of the synergistic role of Curcumin along with ulinastatin (Figure 3) the inhibition of HCT-116 cell migration and invasion occurred [70]. The synergism of Curcumin and ulinastatin was also evaluated in mouse model through dynamically tracking the development of tumor and its therapeutic responses by bioluminescence imaging. A prolonged survival of tumor-bearing mice those treated with the combined agents (Curcumin and ulinastatin) was noticed.

Besides the above, Curcumin confirmed its activity to prevent the undesirable fat accumulation in human hepatocarcinoma cells [71]. It is known that NAFLD (Non-alcoholic fatty liver disease) is one of the major metabolic syndromes globally, caused by the accumulation of liver triglycerides (TG). The underlying reason of NAFLD is an imbalance between uptake, synthesis, export, and oxidation of fatty acids. Curcumin demonstrated hypolipidemic effect by suppressing lipid accumulation and TG as well as total cholesterol (TC) levels in oleic acid-induced human HepG2 liver cancer cells. In the first stage, Curcumin enhanced AMPK phosphorylation to stop the anabolism and promote catabolic pathway by up-regulating PPARα and down-regulating the activity SREBP-1c and FAS to reduce hepatic lipogenesis.

Because of low bioavailability and half-life, a small portion of the orally administered Curcumin can reach at the site of action. Therefore, Curcumin metabolites have been assumed to be responsible for its bioactivity. Curcumin glucuronide (Figure 5) was reported as the major metabolite present in the plasma after oral administration of Curcumin in rats [72].

An interesting study was carried out by Nakagawa and co-workers to compare the activity of Curcumin and its major metabolite Curcumin glucuronide (synthetic) on gene expression in HepG2 human liver cancer cell lines *in vitro*. The RT-PCR (Reverse transcription polymerase chain reaction) was used to detect the RNA expression levels. The effect of Curcumin and Curcumin glucuronide on mRNA expression of *ACOX1*, *GSTT1*, *CAT*, and *AREG* genes was studied. IL-8 expression was also evaluated by real time RT-PCR, because Curcumin inhibits IL-8 production.

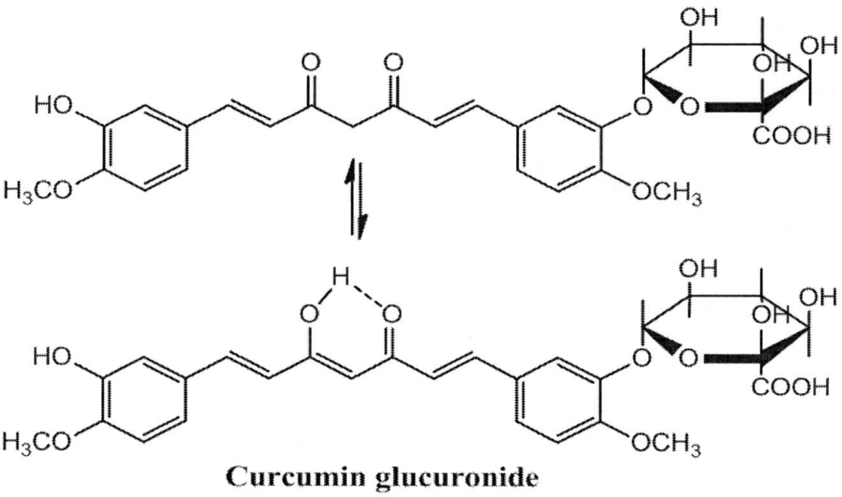

Curcumin glucuronide

Figure 5. Curcumin glucuronide: the major metabolite of Curcumin.

The results showed that the expression of all the tested genes (*ACOX1*, *GSTT1*, *CAT*, *AREG*, and *IL-8*) was significantly decreased by Curcumin treatment, whereas the effect of Curcumin glucuronide was found to be very low.

Curcumin glucuronide down-regulated the expression of *GSTT1* to some extent only. In brief, the *in vitro* cell culture study suggested that Curcumin *per se* was highly active, rather than its major metabolite Curcumin glucuronide.

3.3. Stomach Cancer

Stomach cancer remains one of the major health issues globally. It is the third leading cause of cancer death worldwide with a five-years prevalent of 4.7% in 2012. Anticancer activity of Curcumin on various stomach cancer cells was investigated. It successfully inhibited the cell proliferation of BGC-823 (human stomach adenocarcinoma), MKN-45 (human gastric adenocarcinoma) and SCG-7901 (human gastric cancer) cell lines in a concentration- (1, 5, 10 and 30 μM) and time- (24, 48, 72 and 96 h) dependent manner by inducing apoptosis [73]. Annexin A5 affinity assay (a test to quantify the number of cells undergo apoptosis; the assay uses the protein annexin A5 to tag apoptotic and dead cells, and the numbers are then counted using either flow cytometry or by a fluorescense microscope) confirmed that apoptosis occurred at the dose of 10 and 30 μM when the cells were treated for 24 and 48 h. Total protein analysis revealed that Curcumin up-regulated 33 proteins and down-regulated 42 proteins as determined by spot densitometry. A total of 52 proteins with substantial Mascot scores (Mascot is a software search engine that uses mass spectrometry data to identify proteins from peptide sequence databases) were identified, those were associated with cancer development and progression. The siRNA targeting Chk1 (Checkpoint kinase 1) sensitized the SCG-7901 cells to undergo Curcumin-mediated apoptosis. In another study Curcumin inhibited the fore stomach carcinogenesis induced by benzo[a]pyrene [B(a)P] and micronuclei formation induced by cyclophosphamide in mice [74].

The therapeutic potential of chemotherapy to combat stomach cancer is limited because of chemoresistance which is associated with the expression of NF-κB. Etoposide and doxorubicin are two well-studied anticancer agents with ability to suppress the growth of human gastric cancer SGC-7901 cells in a time- and concentration-dependent manner. The drug synergy of Curcumin in combination with etoposide (Figure 4) or doxorubicin (Figure 4) was studied [75]. Application of Curcumin in addition to etoposide or doxorubicin suppressed the proliferation of SGC-7901 human gastric cancer cell lines. Inhibitory rate was found to be: etoposide *vs.* (etoposide + curcumin), 35% *vs.* 48%, p<0.05 and doxorubicin *vs.* (doxorubicin + curcumin) 33% *vs.* 45%, p<0.05. The results showed that Curcumin intensified the antitumor effects of etoposide and doxorubicin by inhibiting the up-regulation of NF-κB and NF-κB-regulated anti-apoptotic downstream targets Bcl-2 and Bcl- X_L. The combination of Curcumin and the anticancer agents (etoposide or doxorubicin) showed substantial possibility to become an effective therapy for gastric cancer that could synergize the effect of chemotherapeutics and overcome chemoresistance.

The anticancer effect of Curcumin on human gastric carcinoma (AGS), normal gastric epithelial cell line (GES-1) and human gastric cancer cell (MGC-803) was studied. It was found that Curcumin induced apoptosis in the cancer cells and the cytotoxicity was selective toward cancer cells in comparison to normal cells. The molecular mechanism was investigated in human gastric carcinoma (AGS) cell lines. An increased externalization of phosphatidylserine residue was observed by Annexin 5/PI staining along with amended cleavage of procaspase-3, -7, -8 and -9. The study revealed [76] that apoptosis was led by curcumin mediated ER stress and mitochondrial dysfunction as evidenced by expression of CHOP protein, phosphorylation of JNK and repression of SERCA2ATPase, discharge of Cytochrome c, reduction of Bcl-2 and fall of mitochondrial membrane potential. Notably, curcumin reduced cytosolic and ER Ca^{2+}, but augmented mitochondrial Ca^{2+} in the two cell lines which played key role to induce apoptosis leading to cell death. Curcumin inhibited the AGS cell proliferation in a time- and concentration-dependent manner (p<0.05) causing 34% decrease at 5 μmol/L, 51% at 10 μmol/L, and 92% at 25 μmol/L after 96 hours of treatment. It was interesting to note that when curcumin (10 μmol/L) was removed after a 24 hours exposure, the growth pattern of curcumin-treated AGS cells was similar to that of control cells, suggesting reversibility of curcumin on the progression of AGS cells [77]. The combined therapy of Curcumin and 5-fluorouracil (5FU, a pyrimidine analog; it is a suicide inhibitor and works through irreversible inhibition of thymidylate synthase, Figure 4) inhibited the AGS cell proliferation considerably in comparison to either Curcumin or 5-FU monotherapy suggesting the synergistic effect of Curcumin with 5-FU against AGS human gastric cancer cells. It was also found that 96 hours administration of Curcumin (10 μmol/L) in AGS gastric cancer cells, the G2/M phase fraction of the Curcumin treated cells was 60.5% in comparison to 22.0% of the control group, suggesting a G2/M block by Curcumin.

Multidrug resistance (MDR) is a severe problem in cancer chemotherapy. It is often related with the overexpression of ATP-dependent drug efflux proteins belonging to the superfamily of ATP-binding cassette (ABC) transporters namely (i) P-glycoprotein (P-gp, 170 kDa) encoded by the *MDR1* gene and (ii) multidrug resistance-associated protein-1 (MRP-1, 190 kDa) encoded by the *MRP-1* gene. These proteins bind to and transport various structurally unrelated compounds to maintain their intracellular concentrations below cytotoxic levels [78, 79].

Vincristine (brand name, Oncovin, abbreviation: VCR, Figure 4) is a *vinca* alkaloid isolated from the plant *Cantharanthus roseus*. It is a coupled alkaloid of vindoline and cantharanthine, biosynthesized in the plant. Being a potent mitotic inhibitor it is one of the frontline cancer drugs and belongs to WHO's list of essential medicines [80]. The ability of Curcumin to act as a chemosensitizer to sensitize the vincristine (drug) resistant human gastric cancer cells SGC7901/VCR to undergo apoptosis was studied [81]. It increased the sensitivity of SGC7901/VCR cells to vincristine consistently with an increase in intracellular drug concentration by decreasing P-gp function and expression. It is known that P-glycoprotein (P-gp) plays an important role to prevent cell death not only by removing (efflxing) drugs from the cell, but also by inhibiting the activation of proteases associated to initiate (caspase-8) [82] and to execute (caspase-3) apoptotic signaling [82, 83]. Treatment by Curcumin on drug-resistant SGC7901/VCR cells stimulated vincristine-induced caspase-3 activation. P-gp was up-regulated in SGC7901/VCR cells, whereas it was suppressed, at least to some extent, after a 24 hours treatment with Curcumin (10 μmol/L). Resistant cells treated with 1 μmol/L vincristine itself showed 77% lower levels of caspase-3 activation relative to SGC7901 cells, but the activation of caspase-3 in the resistant cell line increased by 44% when cells were treated with vincristine accompanied by Curcumin. Taken together, Curcumin reversed the MDR of the human gastric carcinoma SGC7901/VCR cell line and it could be considered as a promising chemosensitizer of MDR in gastric cancer.

N-nitroso-*N*-methylurea (NMU) is a strong carcinogen, mutagen, and teratogen. It holds the potential to alkylate the nucleobases in nucleic acids by transferring its methyl group, which eventually leads to AT:GC transition mutations. Curcumin treatment on NMU and saturated sodium chloride-induced gastric cancer in male Wistar rats was investigated [84]. At the initiation period Curcumin successfully reduced the gastric cancer through down-regulation of phosphorylated IκBα and 8-OHdG expressions. Besides the above, Curcumin successfully demonstrated its potential as a chemopreventive agent in Phase I clinical trial in patients with high-risk or pre-malignant lesions of gastric cancer [85].

3.4. Colorectal Cancer (Colon Cancer)

Colorectal cancer is the fourth leading cause of cancer-related mortality worldwide in 2012 with a five-years prevalent of 10.9%. The molecular intricacies of colon tumors are not fully understood. *In vitro* studies in human colorectal carcinoma HCT-116 cell line [86] showed the overexpression of a few histone demethylases such as JMJD2A, JMJD2B and JMJD2C but not JMJD2D. Moreover, despite of close homology of JMJD2A-C, their intracellular localizations were different. JMJD2A was mainly localized in cytoplasm and nucleus, JMJD2B preferred to be localized in nucleus only whereas JMJD2C was strongly attached with chromatin. The protein JMJD2C (also known as KDM4C) played crucial roles to develop tumor (HCT-116 cells) by complex formation with β-catenin (an oncoprotein) and promoting its up-regulation. JMJD2C also helped to up-regulate the growth stimulatory proteins FRA1, Cyclin D1 and survival factor Bcl-2. Curcumin exhibited its potential to reduce the activity of JMJD2 enzymes through down-regulation. It was proposed that Curcumin induced sustained activation of JNK, which in turn stimulated apoptosis as a result of inhibition of NFkB transcriptional activity in human colorectal carcinoma (HCT-116) cell line [87].

Later, the same authors reported that it was not essential for Curcumin to inhibit NF-κB for its anti-apoptotic effects rather other unidentified regulators [88] might be involved in cell death process. A study carried out by Wang et al. [89] revealed that neurotensin (an intestinal hormone that was potently released by fat ingestion) acted *via* the native high-affinity neurotensin receptor (NTR) increased the secretion and up-regulation of IL-8 in a concentration- and time-dependent manner. This activation implicated Ca^{2+}-dependent protein kinase C, extracellular signal-regulated kinase-dependent activator protein-1, and extracellular signal-regulated kinase-independent nuclear factor-κB (Ca^{2+}/PKC, ERK/ AP-1, and NF-κB) pathways. These effects eventually enhanced the HCT-116 cell proliferation and migration. Curcumin successfully inhibited gastrointestinal hormone (e.g., neurotensin)-induced chemokine up-regulation and subsequent cell migration. It is known that the enzyme DNAtopoisomerase II alpha (TOP2A) is upregulated in several cancers and acts on RNApolymerase II transcription on chromatin templates. On the other hand, CTCF (also known as 11-zinc finger protein or CCCTC-binding factor, a multifunctional transcription factor) recruits the largest subunit of RNA polymerase II (LS Pol II) and this recruitment of LS Pol II is more pronounced in proliferating cells than in fully differentiated cells. As expression of imprinted genes is often altered in tumors, the therapeutic effect of Curcumin on transcription of the imprinted *H19* gene was investigated [90] in HCT 116 and another human colon adenocarcinoma (SW 620) cell lines. It was concluded that Curcumin down-regulated the TOP2A and subsequently inhibited RNA polymerase II-dependent transcription and eventually - gene transcription was inhibited.

Curcumin inhibited the proteasome and induced apoptosis in both HCT-116 and metastatic SW480 human colon adenocarcinoma cell lines [91]. This study confirmed proteasome as an important cellular target of Curcumin. *In silico* docking studies between proteasome and Curcumin showed that two carbonyl carbons of the Curcumin (Figure 1) were highly susceptible to a nucleophilic attack by the hydroxyl group of the *N*-terminal threonine of the proteasomal chymotrypsin-like (CT-like) subunit. As a result, Curcumin inhibited the proteasome activity in human colon cancer HCT-116 and SW480 cell lines which directed to accumulation of ubiquitinated proteins, several proteasome target proteins, and subsequent induction of apoptosis *in vitro*. The effect was confirmed in animal model through intragastric administration of Curcumin to ICR SCID mice bearing xenografts of colon cancer HCT-116 cells. The experiment resulted in significant inhibition of tumor growth because of proteasomal inhibition which repressed cell proliferation and stimulated cell death *via* apoptosis. It was reported that only 3–5% of all colorectal cancers are due to hereditary genetic defects and up to 25% of patients might have some degree of familiarity for this disease whereas majority of colorectal cancers take place in an erratic fashion without any documented family history. In addition to genetic instability phenotypes such as chromosomal and microsatellite instability, epigenetic alterations that include DNA methylation modifications, histone alterations and variations in miRNA expression might be responsible for the initiation and progression of increasing incidences of colorectal cancers [92, 93]. The effect of Curcumin on DNA methylation of three colorectal cancer cell lines such as HCT116, HT29 (human colorectal adenocarcinoma) and RKO (human colon cancer) was studied [94]. It was found that Curcumin might exhibit its anti-cancer activity, at least in part, *via* epigenetic modulation of DNA methylation changed only in a subset of genes those were distinct from the generalized genomic hypomethylation related with amplified genomic instability in colorectal cancer cells.

Autophagocytosis (or Autophagy, in Greek: *auto* means *self* and *phagein* means *to eat*) is a basic catabolic mechanism which involves the degradation of unnecessary or dysfunctional cellular components in cell *via* the actions of lysosomes. The breakdown of cellular components promotes cellular survival during starvation by maintaining cellular energy levels. Depending upon the state of the disease, autophagy may be a response to stress that promote survival whereas in other cases it appears to promote morbidity or cell death [95, 96].

A study carried out by Mosieniak et al. with HCT-116 cell lines concluded that despite of its low bioavailability, Curcumin could demonstrate good anticancer activity because of cellular senescence of the cancer cells [97]. It was reported that the senescence of cancer and normal cells contained many common features and the senescence of HCT116 cells was correlated with the induction of autophagy. In the case of p53+/+ HCT116 cells, overexpression of the p53 and p21 proteins was observed whereas p53-independent induction of p21 was observed in p53-/- HCT116 cells. The correlation between autophagy and senescence was established by electron microscopy observations of autophagosomes, LC3-II up-regulation, punctue staining of LC3 and increased content of acidic vacuoles in the curcumin-treated cells. However, inhibition of autophagy, due to the reduced expression of Autophagy protein 5 (ATG5) by RNAi reduced the number of senescent cells promoted by curcumin, but did not lead to increased cell death. Another study targeted doublecortin-like kinase 1 (DCLK1), a cancer stem cell marker, to enhance anticancer activity of Curcumin. At optimum concentrations, curcumin significantly decreased expression levels of stem cell markers (DCLK1/CD44/ALDHA1/Lgr5/Nanog) in three-dimensional spheroid cultures and tumor xenograft models derived from colon cancer cells. However, Curcumin surprisingly induced proliferation and autophagic survival of a subset of DCLKl-positive cancer stem cells [98].

Conversely, the combination of DCLK1-siRNA and Curcumin could intensely reverse the phenotype of cancer stem cells. The RNAi-mediated silencing of DCLK1 activated Curcumin-induced apoptotic cell death of colon cancer cells *in vitro* and *in vivo*.

Cortactin (cortical actin binding protein CTTN, a monomeric protein located in the cytoplasm of cells), encoded by the *CTTN/EMS1* gene, is a v-Src substrate localized with cortical actin at the plasma membrane and is up-regulated in several types of cancer [99]. The phosphorylated form of cortactin (pTyr421) plays major role in cancer cell migration and invasion. It was shown that pTyr421-cortactin was up-regulated in colon cancer.

Curcumin interacted with PTPN1 tyrosine phosphatases to rise its efficacy leading to dephosphorylation of pTyr421-CTTN. Curcumin considerably reduced the pTyr421-CTTN in

HCT116 cells and SW480 (adenocarcinoma of the colon) cells, but was ineffective in HT-29 (human colorectal adenocarcinoma) cells.

Altogether, Curcumin modulated the activity of PTPN1 phosphatase to reduce cortactin phosphorylation and interaction with CTNND1, and finally to reduce colon cancer cell migration [100]. Curcumin activated MAPKs including Erk1/2 and JNK and inhibited phosphatases 2A (PP2A) and 5 (PP5). Up-regulation of MAPK cascade induce ROS which ultimately led to p53-independent apoptosis in cancer cells [101].

Treatment with Curcumin destroyed wild-type p53 HCT-116 cells and mutant p53 HT-29 cells in a concentration- and time-dependent fashion. Curcumin treatment also exhibited equivalent cytotoxic effect in $p53^{+/+}$ and $p53^{-/-}$ HCT-116 cells, validating that curcumin-induced cytotoxicity was independent of p53 status. Therefore, Curcumin holds the therapeutic potential to combat with the colorectal tumors those are resistant to conventional chemotherapy due to defects in p53 expression or function [102].

Curcumin treatment on other colorectal cancer cell lines was also investigated. Curcumin repressed the proliferation of HCT-15 (human colorectal adenocarcinoma) cells by inducing apoptosis in a time- and concentration-dependent manner [103]. The apoptotic pathway was proposed by activation of caspase-3, down-regulation of pre-mRNA processing factor 4B (PRP4B) and generation of ROS. Curcumin-induced inhibition of proliferation in HT-29 (human colon adenocarcinoma) and Caco-2 (heterogeneous human epithelial colorectal adenocarcinoma) proceeded by repression of EGFR [104].

The process was initiated by the interruption of the ERK signal pathway by down-regulating ERK and subsequently its activity was reduced. Accordingly the transcription factor early growth response-1 (Egr-1) was suppressed and Egr trans-activity was reduced which finally down-regulated the EGFR expression leading to inhibition of colon cancers (HT-29 and Caco-2) cell proliferation.

Treatment with Curcumin could successfully inhibited the proliferation of human colon cancer (COLO 205) cells through apoptosis, in concentration- and time-dependent manner, by the generation of Ca^{2+} and ROS, followed by attenuation of the levels of mitochondria membrane potential and finally the activation of caspase-3 [105].

The same research group also reported that Curcumin attenuated the N-acetyltransferase (NAT) activity in a concentration-dependent manner in COLO 205 cells. Moreover Curcumin treatment also reduced the DNA adduct formation and down-regulated gene (NAT1) mRNA expression [106].

The treatment of colorectal cancer is challenging because of drug resistance. In particular, more than 15% patients are found to be resistant to 5-Fluorouracil (5-FU, Figure 4) derived chemotherapeutic agents. Accordingly, the colorectal tumor relapses in case of more than 50% patients. Curcumin demonstrated promising chemosensitizing activity to sensitize DNA mismatch repair (MMR)-proficient 5-FU-resistant colon cancer cells HCT116R, HCT116+ch3R (complemented with chromosome 3) in high density 3D culture which resulted in improved fragmentation of colonospheres, increased apoptosis and related growth inhibition [107]. Curcumin drawn considerable interest to serve as radiosensitizer in colorectal cancer radiotherapy. Radio-resistance can be facilitated by constitutively active pro-survival signaling pathways or by inducible/acquired mechanisms in response to radiation therapy. The NF-κB activation was characterized as a mechanism of inducible radio-resistance in colorectal cancer (HCT116, HT29, and SW620) cells.

For the Curcumin-pretreated cells the resistance can be successfully overcome and better radiotherapeutic effect can be achieved [108]. Curcumin inhibited the proliferation and the post-irradiation clonogenic survival of colorectal cancer cells.

It also down-regulated the radiation-induced NF-κB activation through inhibition of radiation-induced phosphorylation, repressing NF-κB-regulated gene products (Bcl-2, Bcl-x$_L$, inhibitor of apoptosis protein-2, cyclooxygenase-2, and cyclin D1) and inhibition of Akt phosphorylation.

Curcumin showed synergistic activity with various drugs/compounds against colorectal cancer cell lines. This activity can be summarized as shown in Table 3.

Apart from the above discussion, the Phase I trial of oral Curcumin was carried out which advocated for its Phase II evaluation in the prevention or treatment of cancers outside the gastrointestinal tract [116]. A recent clinical pilot study aimed to quantify levels of curcuminoids in colorectal mucosa of patients after administration of oral curcumin [117] yielded promising results and recommended the regimen as safe, and patients support its use in long-term trials.

Table 3. Synergistic effect of Curcumin against colorectal cancer

Cell (s)	Drug/Compound[*]	Mechanism of action	Reference
HT-29	5-FU	Inhibition of COX-2 expression.	[109]
HCT116 and HCT116+ch3 (complemented with chromosome 3)	5-FU	Inhibition of NF-κB and Src protein kinase signaling pathways.	[110]
HT-29	Ritanserin	Suppression of the serotonin 5-HT$_{2A}$ receptor.	[111]
Chemo-resistant HCT-116 and HT-29	Dasatinib	Down-regulation of CD133, CD44, CD166 and ALDH.	[112]
HCT-116	Dasatinib	Not known.	[113]
HCT-116	Resveratrol	Inhibition of constitutive activation of EGFR and its family members and IGF-1R.	[114]
HT-29, IEC-18-K-ras, Caco-2 and SW-480	Celecoxib	Inhibition of COX-2 and other non-COX-2 pathways.	[115]

[*]See Figure 4.

3.5. Breast Cancer

The incidence of breast cancer (both sexes) was second highest among all cancers (11.9%) and it was the leading cause of mortality due to cancer among women worldwide (fifth for both genders) in 2012 [39]. Several research laboratories around the world have been engaged to investigate the pharmacological potential of Curcumin against different types of breast cancer. Curcumin could successfully inhibit the proliferation of human breast cancer MDA-MB-435 cells in a concentration- and time-dependent manner by accumulating the cells in the G_1 phase of the cell cycle. The overexpression of *EZH2* in human breast cancer MDA-MB-435 cells caused poor prognosis in this type of cancer. The underlying molecular mechanism of Curcumin treatment was explained by the activation of the MAPK signaling pathway. Three major members of the MAPK family, the p38 kinase, JNK and ERK were stimulated to down-regulate the enhancer of zeste homolog 2 (*EZH2*) gene overexpression leading to proliferation of the cancer cells [118]. Activated cancer-associated fibroblasts (CAFs) or myofibroblasts facilitate the growth of tumor as well as develop drug-resistance in human breast cancer. Hence effective therapeutic regimen should be able to inhibit the paracrine effects of these supportive cells. Treatment with Curcumin on patient-derived primary breast CAF cells overexpressed p16^{INK4A} and other tumor suppressor proteins while inactivated the JAK2/STAT3 pathway. This repressed the alpha-smooth muscle actin (α-SMA) and consequently the cell migration/invasion was reduced [119]. Curcumin also down-regulated Lamin B1 and initiated DNA damage-independent senescence in proliferating but not inactive breast stromal fibroblasts. Curcumin-induced senescence was p16^{INK4A}-dependent and occurred with no associated inflammatory secretory phenotype.

Approximately 15% of all breast cancers are triple-negative breast cancer (TNBC). In TNBC, the reoccurrence of tumor rate is high with poor prognosis and low survival rate.

TNBC is characterized by the lack expression of progesterone receptor (PR), estrogen receptor (ER) and epidermal growth factor receptor 2 (HER2/cerbB2/EGFR2) expression [120, 121]. Therefore, TNBC lacks effective targeted therapies. The only possible therapeutic option in the adjuvant or metastatic situation is chemotherapy but most unfortunately TNBC is often resistant to standard chemotherapeutic regimens. Consequently, TNBC has the worst prognosis and survival rate of all breast cancer subtypes. Curcumin demonstrated its ability to inhibit the proliferation of MDA-MB-231 TNBC cells inducing apoptosis *in vitro* by inhibiting the EGFR signaling pathway [122]. The level of apoptosis of the curcumin-treated (30 μmol/mL) group (26.34%) was significantly different from that of the control group (2.76%). All these findings suggest that further studies with Curcumin are required, particularly in this subset of breast cancer patients, for those proper treatment opportunities are very limited. The anti-breast cancer effect of Curcumin was also evaluated with three other TNBC cells such as MDA-MB-468 (MDA468), HCC1937, and HCC1806 by Nahta and co-workers [123]. Besides these, HER2-overexpressing SKBR3 cells, ERα (+) MCF7 human breast cancer cells, and non-transformed mammary epithelial MCF12A cell lines were also evaluated with Curcumin. The molecular mechanism was described by the DNA damage in TNBC cells along with phosphorylation, increased expression, and cytoplasmic retention of the BRCA1 protein. Moreover, Curcumin induced apoptosis and anchorage-independent cell growth (which is considered as a hall mark in cancer biology) and subsequent migration of TNBC cells. In case of non-transformed mammary epithelial MCF12A cells apoptosis and BRCA1 protein modulation were not observed which might be considered as target specificity of curcumin toward TNBC cells.

To evaluate the anticancer effect of the dietary antioxidant Curcumin on mammary cells which are resistant to oxidative damage, human breast cancer cells ZR-75-1 were treated with Curcumin and $CuSO_4$ in order to assess cell proliferation and GGTP (γ-glutamyltranspeptidase) activity. Curcumin demonstrated cytotoxicity toward ZR-75-1 cells and down-regulated GGTP activity in a concentration-dependent manner. It induced apoptosis and exhibited antioxidant effect only on the copper-oxidized cells. Taken together, Curcumin inhibited the proliferation of human breast cancer ZR-75-1 cells under oxidative stress through apoptosis [124]. In another study it was revealed that Curcumin induced anti-proliferative effect on two human breast cancer cell lines (MDA-MB-231 and BT-483) in a concentration- and time-dependent manner *via* apoptosis [124]. The results showed that the expression of Cyclin D1 was down-regulated in MDA-MB-231 cells whereas CDK4 expression was down-regulated in BT-483 breast cancer cells. On the other hand, MMP1 mRNA expression was significantly down-regulated in both the breast cancer cells. Altogether it was concluded that Curcumin-induced anti-proliferative effect was due to suppression of NFκB inducing genes [125]. To investigate whether Curcumin-induced cell proliferation and apoptosis in human breast cancer MDA-MB-231 cell lines were associated with down-regulation of *Notch1* gene expression as well as NF-κB suppression, the mRNA and protein expression of *Notch1* and NF-κB were measured by RT-PCR and Western blot [126]. The results showed that the mRNA and protein levels of *Notch1* and NF-κB were reduced considerably in concentration- and time-dependent manner ($P < 0.05$). From this observation it was concluded that the Notch-1 signaling pathway was mechanistically linked with NF-κB activity during curcumin-induced inhibition of cell growth and cell death through apoptosis in human breast cancer MDA-MB-231 cell lines.

It was also supported that Curcumin-induced apoptosis in human breast cancer MCF-7 cells was accompanied by an increase in p53 level as well as its DNA-binding activity followed by Bax expression at the protein level [127].

Human epidermal growth factor receptor 2 (*HER2* or *HER2/neu*) is an oncogene and its overexpression plays a key role in the growth and progression of certain aggressive type of breast cancers with higher relapse rate, and increased mortality. It has become an important biomarker and therapeutic target of about 20-30% of breast cancer patients [128]. HER-2 is an important oncoprotein overexpressed in about 15-25% of breast cancers. It was hypothesized that the ability of curcumin to down-regulate HER-2 oncoprotein and inhibit the signal transduction pathway of PI3K/Akt, MAPK, and NF-κB activation may be important in the treatment of HER-2-overexpressed breast cancer. The therapeutic potential of Curcumin to down-regulate HER-2 oncoprotein was investigated in five human breast cancer cells: MCF-7, MDA-MB-231, MCF-10A, BT-474, and SK-BR-3-hr (a herceptin resistant strain from SK-BR-3) *in vitro*. The HER-2-overexpressed BT-474 xenograft model was used for *in vivo* validation of Curcumin on HER-2-overexpressed breast cancer. Curcumin successfully reduced the cell proliferation in all the five tested breast cancer cell lines. The Western blot analysis showed that the phosphorylation of Akt, MAPK, and expression of NF-κB were reduced in BT-474 cells, but not in SK-BR-3-hr cells, after treatment with herceptin. When treated with curcumin, the HER-2 oncoprotein, phosphorylation of Akt, MAPK and expression of NF-κB were decreased in both BT-474 and SK-BR-3-hr cells. In the BT-474 xenograft model, though not as much as herceptin, Curcumin effectually reduced the tumor size [129].

Circulating tumor cells (CTC) are present into the vasculature from a primary tumor and flow in the bloodstream. Therefore, CTCs can be considered as seeds for subsequent growth of additional tumors (metastasis) in distant organs, initiating a mechanism that is responsible for the vast majority of cancer-related deaths [130]. As stated earlier, invasion and metastasis are two serious problems for the prevention/treatment of cancer. The properties of circulating tumor cells (CTC) and cancer stem-like cells (CSC) are related with distant metastasis, but the mechanisms through which CSCs promote metastasis are not clear. It was reported that breast cancer cell lines with more stem-like properties display higher levels of microtentacles

(McTN), a type of tubulin-based protrusion of the plasma cell membrane that forms on detached or suspended cells and aid in cell reattachment. Curcumin promptly quenched McTN in breast CSC, preventing reattachment from suspension.

Overall, a model in which breast CSCs with cytoskeletal alterations that promote McTNs can mediate attachment and metastasis but might be targeted by Curcumin as an anti-metastatic strategy [131]. Chronic inflammation is a key risk factor for the growth and metastatic development of cancer. Curcumin inhibited the expression of the proinflammatory cytokines CXCL1 and -2 to reduce breast and prostate cancer metastases. From the microarray miRNA expression analysis it was found that Curcumin modulated the expression of a series of miRNAs, including up-regulation of miR181b, in metastatic breast cancer MDA-MB-231 cells where miR181b down-regulated the proinflammatory cytokines CXCL1 and -2 through a direct binding to their 3'-UTR. Curcumin-induced up-regulation of miR181b in metastatic breast cancer cells inhibited metastasis formation *in vivo* in immune-deficient mice [132]. Another study in this field suggested that metastatic development in human mammary epithelial carcinoma MCF-7 cells was inhibited by Curcumin *via* the suppression of urokinase-type plasminogen activator by NF-κB signaling pathways [133].

MMP-9 is a major factor in cancer cell invasion. An invasion-related study in MCF-7 human breast cancer cells [134] supported that Curcumin suppressed the TPA-induced MMP-9 expression and subsequent cell invasion.

The molecular mechanism involved Curcumin-induced inhibition of PKCα-dependent MMP-expression, down-regulation of NF-κB and reduction of AP-1 activation i.e. repression of the PKCα, MAPK and NF-κB/AP-1 pathway in MCF-7 cells.

It has been found that breast cancer is often associated with obesity. Most probably the relation between these two factors is mediated by adipokines. Visfatin [Nicotinamide phosphoribosyltransferase (NAmPRTase or Nampt) also known as pre-B-cell colony-enhancing factor 1 (PBEF1)] is an adipokine, that is localized to the bloodstream and has various functions. The protein visfatin has recently been shown to be related to the development and progression of breast cancer.

Consequently, suppression of the gene *visfatin* might be a novel strategy to fight against breast cancer. The influence of Curcumin on *visfatin* gene suppression was investigated [135]. It was found that the mRNA and protein levels of *visfatin* were down-regulated by Curcumin in human breast cancer MDA-MB-231, MDA-MB-468, and MCF-7 cell lines. In addition, the activity of constitutive nuclear factor (NF)-κB was reduced.

Taken together, *visfatin* could enhance the invasion of breast cancer cells which was down-regulated by Curcumin. Furthermore, *visfatin* knockdown by siRNA led to the reduction of cancer cell invasion. Curcumin treatment could impose anti-migratory activity in human breast cancer MDA-MB-231 cells [136]. It inhibited proliferation and migration by increasing the Bax to Bcl-2 ratio and decreasing NF-κBp65 expression. Integrin (α6β4) is a laminin adhesion receptor with an established role in the invasion and migration of cancer cells. Curcumin successfully decreased the integrin (α6β4)-dependent breast cancer cell motility and invasion in a dose-dependent manner without affecting apoptosis in MDA-MB-435/β4 (β$_4$-integrin transfectants) and MDA-MB-231 breast cancer cell lines [137].

Maspin (mammary serine protease inhibitor) can suppress tumor growth and metastasis *in vivo* and tumor cell motility and invasion *in vitro* in breast cancer. The maspin expression in Curcumin-treated MCF-7 (wild type p53) at transcription and translation levels was analyzed by RT-PCR, immunofluorescence, and Western blotting.

The results showed a correlation of maspin expression with p53 and Bcl-2 levels. Curcumin inhibited cell proliferation by inducing apoptosis and up-regulation of *maspin* gene expression was observed in MCF-7 cells.

These findings were further correlated with the up-regulation of p53 protein and down-regulation of Bcl-2, suggesting maspin mediated apoptosis in MCF-7 cancer cells [138]. The chemopreventive activity of Curcumin in transformed breast cells was investigated [139]. Curcumin inhibited H-ras-induced invasive phenotype in MCF10A human breast epithelial cells (H-ras MCF10A); repressed MMP-2 and exerted cytotoxic effect on H-ras MCF10A cells in concentration-dependent manner. The apoptotic cell death involved significant down-regulation of Bcl-2 and up-regulation of Bax.

Curcumin treatment resulted in the generation of ROS in H-ras MCF10A cells. In brief, the results supported that curcumin inhibited invasion and induced apoptosis in the transformed breast cancer H-ras MCF10A cells.

Drug-synergy has also been demonstrated by Curcumin with several other drugs against breast cancer cell lines. A brief description is outlined below (Table 4):

Table 4. Synergistic effect of Curcumin against breast cancer

Cell (s)	Drug/Compound*	Mechanism of action	Reference
MCF-7	LY290042 (PI3K inhibitor, Figure 4)	Apoptotic cell death *via* Akt phosphorylation and GSK3β up-regulation	[140]
TNBC cells: MDA-MB-468, MDA-MB- 231, BT-549, and BT-20	Doxorubicin	Inhibition of TGF-β and PI3K/AKT signaling pathways	[141]
MCF-7	Mitomycin C	Inhibition of GRP58-mediated DNA cross-linking through the ERK/p38 MAPK pathway	[142]**
MDA-MB-231	Taxol (Paclitaxel)	Inhibition of paclitaxel-induced activation of NF-κB and potentiation of the growth inhibitory effect of paclitaxel	[143]
MDA-MB-231	Xanthorrhizol	Alteration of mitochondrial transmembrane potential: Apoptosis	[144]

*See Figure 4.
**Curcumin reduces the side effects of mitomycin C.

3.6. Miscellaneous

Aside from the previous discussion, anticancer effect of Curcumin was evaluated for many other types of cancer. Some representative examples are summarized in Table 5.

Conclusion and Future Aspects

Curcumin is a non-toxic, cheap and easily available natural polyphenol with high medicinal and commercial demands. Many costly products can be derived from Curcumin. For example, Curcumin can easily be converted to vanillin through a single-step conversion [172].

However, a huge number of preclinical and early-phase clinical studies undoubtedly confirmed that Curcumin, the golden spice [173] from India, is safe with vast potential of becoming an effective drug for several human diseases including chronic inflammation and cancer. Moreover, the results of clinical trials are under progress in different parts of the world. A serious concern regarding pharmacological application of Curcumin is its poor pharmacokinetics (PK) profile. The bioavailability of Curcumin is low because of poor absorption, rapid elimination and/or low target organ concentration. This is due to the reason that Curcumin is conjugated when it is absorbed through the intestine, consequently free curcumin is present at extremely low level in the target organ.

Moreover, in biological system it is rapidly converted to its metabolites. Nevertheless, Curcumin is non-toxic with a dose of 8g/day is well tolerable and 12g/day may cause minor adverse effects like diarrhea, headache, yellowish stools and rashes etc.

Table 5. Anticancer activity of Curcumin on different types of cancer

Cancer type/Cell	Description/Mechanism of action	Reference
Oral		
SAS and SAS/luc (transfected with *luc* gene)	SAS cancer cell proliferation was greatly inhibited *in vitro* and *in vivo* (xenograft model). Apoptosis: G2/M phase arrest.	[145]
Nasopharyngeal		
Detroit 562 and HONE-1	Inhibition of cell proliferation inducing apoptosis *via* caspase-3-dependent pathway.	[146]
NPC/CNE2	Dark cytotoxicity and photocytotoxicity: Apoptosis	[147]
CNE-2Z	Inhibit cell proliferation by apoptosis. Alters expression of proteins in the ERK-1/2 signaling pathway.	[148]
Oesophageal (Esophageal)		
OE19, OE21, OE33 and KYSE450	Inhibition of cell proliferation *via* non-apoptotic form of cell death. Caspase-3 activation was detected in two out of four cell lines (OE21 and OE33), but was a minor event.	[149]
TE-7, TE-10 (Human esophageal adenocarcinoma) ESO-1 (mouse esophageal adenocarcinoma).	Apoptosis through caspase 3 activation. Down-regulation of Cyclin D1 Down-regulate the expressions of *Notch-1* specific microRNAs, miR-21 and miR-34a, and upregulation of tumor suppressor let-7a miRNA.	[150]
Gallbladder		
GBC-SD	Apoptosis by regulating the ratio of Bcl-2/Bax and activating the expression of cleaved caspase-3.	[151]
HAG-1	G_2/M arrest and apoptosis through multiple mechanisms involving enhanced mitogen-activated protein (MAP) kinase activity, reduced Akt-mTOR activity, and reduced Bcl-2 function.	[152]

Cancer type/Cell	Description/Mechanism of action	Reference
Pancreas		
MIA PaCa-2	Inhibition of cell proliferation inducing apoptosis. Downregulation of the transcription nuclear factor NF-κB and NF-κB-regulated gene products	[153]
BxPC-3 and MIA PaCa-2	Inhibition of cell proliferation inducing apoptosis. Activation of TNFR, CASP 8, CASP3, BID, BAX, and down-regulation of NFκB, NDRG 1, and BCL2L10.	[154]
Larynx		
HEp2	Downregulation MMP-2 expression and activity and expression of integrin receptors, FAK, and MT1-MMP to almost background levels. MMP-2 (but not MMP-9) mRNA expression was abolished.	[155]
Cervix		
KB-V1	Duel modulation of MDR1 expression and Pgp function	[156]
HeLa	Down-regulate HPV18 transcription as well as the AP-1 binding activity. Reverse the expression dynamics of c-fos and fra-1.	[157]
Ovary		
HEY, OVCA429, OCC1, SKOV3	Inhibition of cell proliferation inducing p53-independent apoptosis that involved p38 MAPK activation, ablation of prosurvival Akt signaling, and reduced expression of the antiapoptotic proteins Bcl-2 and surviving.	[158]
OVCA 420 and OVCA 429	Suppression of JAK-STAT signaling *via* activation of PIAS-3, thus attenuating STAT-3 phosphorylation and tumor cell growth.	[159]
Prostate		
LNCaP and PC-3	Apoptosis through Bax translocation to mitochondria and caspase activation.	[160]
DU145 and PC-3	Tumor necrosis factor-related apoptosis-inducing ligand (TRAIL/Apo2L)-induced apoptosis by inhibiting nuclear factor (NF)-κB.	[161]
Testis		
NTera-2	Dose-dependently induced apoptosis of NTera-2 cells by reducing FasL expression and Bcl-2-to-Bax ratio, and activating caspase-9, -8 and -3. Repression of AP transcription factor AP-2γ.	[162]
Kidney		
Caki	Induced apoptosis through the production of ROS, and the down-regulation of Bcl-xL and inhibitor of apoptosis protein (IAP) in Caki cells. Enhanced dual PI3K/Akt and mTOR inhibitor NVP-BEZ235-induced apoptosis in human renal carcinoma Caki cells through down-regulation of p53-dependent Bcl-2 expression and inhibition of Mcl-1 protein stability.	[163]
ACHN	Induced apoptosis. Up-regulation of IκB, down-regulation of NF-κB, and modulationof the expression of the apoptosis genes Bcl-2/Bax.	[164]

Table 5. (Continued)

Cancer type/Cell	Description/Mechanism of action	Reference
Brain		
Glioma	Induced apoptosis by inhibition of SHH/GLI1 signaling pathway.	[165]
Thyroid		
FTC-133	FTC-133 cell invasion was inhibited *via* down-regulation of PI3K/Akt signaling pathway.	[166]
K1	Metastasis of K1 papillary thyroid cancer cells was inhibited *via* modulating E-cadherin and matrix metalloproteinase-9 expression.	[167]
Multiple Myeloma		
MM	Constitutive and IL-6-inducible STAT3 phosphorylation was inhibited.	[168]
MM	Constitutive activation of nuclear factor-κB and IκBα kinase in human multiple myeloma cells was down-regulated, leading to suppression of proliferation and induction of apoptosis.	[169]
Leukaemia		
THP-1	Apoptosis *via* simultaneously targeting Akt/mTOR and RAF/MEK/ERK survival signaling pathways.	[170]
JURKAT	Caspase mediated apoptosis by disrupting the redox balance.	[171]

On the other hand, curcumin demonstrated diverse anticancer properties *in vitro*, *ex vivo* and *in vivo* as well as in clinical trials by inducing a variety of biological pathways involved in apoptosis, tumor proliferation, chemoprevention, chemo- and radiosensitization, tumor invasion, metastasis and angiogenesis. Curcumin can be an effective adjunct in treating solid organ tumors due to its properties of regulating oncogenes like *p53*, *egr-1*, *c-myc*, *Bcl- X_L*, etc.; transcription factors like NF-kB, STAT-3, β-catenin and AP-1; growth factors (EGF, PDGF, and VEGF); protein kinases like MAPK, Cyclin D1, CDKs, Akt, PKC; and enzymes like COX, LOX, MMP and many others. Based on its huge therapeutic aspects several active investigations are going on to overcome the ADME-related drawbacks by introducing new and novel formulation and route of administration to achieve the highest therapeutic level. It is highly expected that curcumin will become an effective cancer drug in future with novel formulation and/or unique route of administration.

Acknowledgments

The author is thankful to the Kleberg Foundation of Texas and the University of Texas-Pan American.

References

[1]   http://www.nutraceuticalsworld.com/contents/view_health-e-insights/2011-10-28/an-interview-with-dr-stephen-defelice/ (Access date: December 29, 2013).

[2]   *Health Canada policy paper.* Therapeutic Products Programme and the Food Directorate from the Health Protection Branch. Nutraceuticals/Functional Foods and Health Claims on Foods, archived on June 24, 2013 (http://www.hc-sc.gc.ca/fn-an/alt_ formats/hpfb-dgpsa/pdf/label-etiquet/nutra-funct_foods-nutra-fonct_aliment-eng.pdf) (Access date: December 29, 2013).

[3]   Advances in experimental medicine and biology (Vol. 595). In: *The Molecular Target and Therapeutic Uses of Curcumin in Health and Disease*, Aggarwal, B. B.; Surh, Y. J.; Shishodia, S. Eds.; Springer: New York, NY, US, 2007.

[4]   Padhye, S.; Chavan, D.; Pandey, S.; Deshpande, J.; Swamy, K. V.; Sarkar, F. H. Perspectives on chemopreventive and therapeutic potential of curcumin analogs in medicinal chemistry. *Mini. Rev. Med. Chem.* 2010, 10, 372-387.

[5]   Epstein, J.; Sanderson, I. R.; MacDonald, T. T. Curcumin as a therapeutic agent: the evidence from in vitro, animal and human studies. *Brit. J. Nutr.* 2010, 103, 1545-1557

[6]   http://www.accessdata.fda.gov/scripts/fcn/fcnNavigation.cfm?filter=turmericandsort Column=andrpt=grasListing (Access date: December 30, 2013).

[7]   Aggarwal, B. B.; Sundaram, C.; Malani, N.; Ichikawa, H. Curcumin: The Indian solid gold. *Adv. Exp. Med. Biol.* 2007, 595, 1-75.

[8]   Spices Board of India. Ministry of Commerce and Industry. Available online: http://www.indianspices.com (Access date: December 30, 2013).

[9]   Ploto, A. *Turmeric: Post-Production Management for Improved Market Access for Herbs and Spices-Turmeric*; Food and Agriculture Organization of the United Nations (FAO): Rome, Italy, 2003.

[10]   Basnet, P.; Skalko-Basnet, N. Curcumin: An anti-inflammatory molecule from a curry spice on the path to cancer treatment. *Molecules*, 2011, 16, 4567-4598.

[11]   World Health Organization. Rhizoma curcumae longae. In: *WHO Monographs on Selected Medicinal Plants*; WHO: Geneva, Switzerland, 1999; Volume 1, pp. 115-124.

[12]   Hatcher, H.; Planalp, R.; Cho, J.; Torti, F. M.; Torti, S. V. Curcumin: From ancient medicine to current clinical trials. *Cell. Mol. Life Sci.* 2008, 65, 1631-1652.

[13]   Salvioli, S.; Sikora, E.; Cooper, E. L.; Franceschi, C. Curcumin in cell death processes: a challenge for CAM of age related pathologies. *Evid. Based Complement. Alternat. Med.* 2007, 4, 181-190.

[14]   Gupta, S. C.; Sung, B.; Kim, J. H.; Prasad, S.; Li, S.; Aggarwal, B. B. Multitargeting by turmeric, the golden spice: From kitchen to clinic. *Mol. Nutr. Food Res.* 2013, 57, 1510-1528.

[15]   Ammon, H. P. T.; Wahl, M. A. Pharmacology of *Curcuma longa. Planta Med.* 1991, 57, 1-7.

[16]   Chattopadhyay, I.; Biswas, K.; Bandyopadhyay, U.; Banerjee, R. K. Turmeric and curcumin: Biological actions and medicinal applications. *Cur. Sci.* 2004, 87, 44-53.

[17]   Goel, A.; Kunnumakkara, A. B.; Aggarwal, B. B. Curcumin as "Curecumin": From kitchen to clinic. *Biochem. Pharmacol.* 2008, 75, 787-809.

[18]   Vogel, H. A.; Pelletier, J. Curcumin-biological and medicinal properties. *J. Pharma.* 1815, 2, 50.

[19]   Gupta, S. C.; Patchva, S.; Koh, W.; Aggarwal, B. B. Discovery of curcumin, a component of the golden spice, and its miraculous biological activities. *Clin. Exp. Pharmacol. Physiol.* 2012, 39, 283-299.

[20]   Vogel, A. *J. de Pharm. et Chim.*, 1842, 3, 20.

[21] Milobedzka, J.; Kostanecki, V.; Lampe, V. Zur Kenntnis des curcumins. *Ber Dtsch. Chem. Ges.* 1910, 43, 2163-2170.

[22] Lampe, V.; Milobedzka, J. Studien uber curcumin. *Ber Dtsch. Chem. Ges.* 1913, 46, 2235-2237.

[23] Roughley, P. J.; Whiting, D. A. Experiments in the biosynthesis of curcumin. *J. Chem. Soc. Perkin Trans.* 1, 1973, 20, 2379-2388.

[24] Payton, F.; Sandusky, P.; Alworth, W. L. NMR study of the solution structure of curcumin. *J. Nat. Prod.* 2007, 70, 143-146.

[25] Advances in experimental medicine and biology (Vol. 595). In: *The Molecular Target and Therapeutic Uses of Curcumin in Health and Disease*, Aggarwal, B. B.; Surh, Y. J.; Shishodia, S. Eds. In: *Curcumin: The Indian solid gold*, Aggarwal, B. B.; Sundaram, C.; Malani, N.; Ichikawa, H.; Springer: New York, NY, US, 2007, pp. 1-75.

[26] http://en.wikipedia.org/wiki/Curcuma (Access date: December 31, 2013).

[27] Loeber, K. C.; Buechner, A. E. Dissertatio inauguralis medica de Curcuma Officinarum Ejusque Genuinis Virtutibus. Præs. A. E. Büchnero, Etc. *Diss Inaug Halae.* 1748, Publisher: Halae Magdeburgicae, Typis Jo. Christiani Hendelii, pp. 28.

[28] National Cancer Institute. Clinical development plan: Curcumin. *J. Cell. Biochem. Suppl.* 1996, 26, 72-85.

[29] Oppenheimer, A. Turmeric (curcumin) in biliary diseases. *Lancet.* 1937, 229, 619-621.

[30] Schraufstatter, E.; Bernt, H. Antibacterial action of curcumin and related compounds. *Nature*, 1949, 164, 456-457.

[31] Chaudhri, K. R. C. Turmeric, haldi or haridra, in eye disease. *Antiseptic*, 1950, 47, 67.

[32] Jiang, T. L.; Salmon, S. E.; Liu, R. M. Activity of camptothecin, harringtonin, cantharidin and curcumae in the human tumor stem cell assay. *Eur. J. Cancer Clin. Oncol.* 1983, 19, 263-270.

[33] Kuttan, R.; Bhanumathy, P.; Nirmala, K.; George, M. C. Potential anticancer activity of turmeric (Curcuma longa). *Cancer Lett.* 1985, 29, 197-202.

[34] http://www.who.int/mediacentre/factsheets/fs297/en (Accessed on July 21, 2014).

[35] http://globocan.iarc.fr/Pages/fact_sheets_cancer.aspx (Accessed on July 21, 2014).

[36] Vogelstein, B.; Kinzler, K. W. Cancer genes and the pathways they control. *Nat. Med.* 2004, 10, 789-799.

[37] Newman, D. J.; Cragg, G. M.; Snader, K. M. Natural products as sources of new drugs over the period 1981-2002. *J. Nat. Prod.*, 2003, 66, 1022-1037.

[38] Hasima, N.; Aggarwal, B. B. Cancer-linked targets modulated by curcumin. *Int. J. Biochem. Mol. Biol.*, 2012, 3, 328-351.

[39] http://globocan.iarc.fr/Pages/fact_sheets_population.aspx (Accessed on July 24, 2014).

[40] Sen, S.; Sharma, H.; Singh, N. Curcumin enhances vinorelbine mediated apoptosis in NSCLC cells by the mitochondrial pathway. *Biochem. Biophys. Res. Commun.* 2005, 331, 1245-1252.

[41] Lev-Ari, S.; Starr, A.; Vexler, A.; Karaush, V.; Loew, V.; Greif, J.; Fenig, E.; Aderka, D.; Ben-Yosef, R. Inhibition of pancreatic and lung adenocarcinoma cell survival by curcumin is associated with increased apoptosis, down-regulation of COX-2 and EGFR and inhibition of Erk1/2 activity. *Anticancer Res.* 2006, 26, 4423-4430.

[42] Radhakrishna Pillai, G.; Srivastava, A. S.; Hassanein, T. I.; Chauhan, D. P.; Carrier, E. Induction of apoptosis in human lung cancer cells by curcumin. *Cancer Lett.* 2004, 208, 163-170.

[43] Shankar, S.; Srivastava, R. K. Bax and Bak genes are essential for maximum apoptotic response by curcumin, a polyphenolic compound and cancer chemopreventive agent derived from turmeric, *Curcuma longa*. *Carcinogenesis*, 2007, 28, 1277-1286.

[44] Chanvorachote, P.; Pongrakhananon, V.; Wannachaiyasit, S.; Luanpitpong, S.; Rojanasakul, Y.; Nimmannit, U. Curcumin Sensitizes Lung Cancer Cells to Cisplatin-Induced Apoptosis Through Superoxide Anion-Mediated Bcl-2 Degradation. *Cancer Invest.* 2009, 27, 624-635.

[45] Biswas, S. K.; McClure, D.; Jimenez, L. A.; Megson, I. L.; Rahman, I. Curcumin induces glutathione biosynthesis and inhibits NF-kappaB activation and interleukin-8 release in alveolar epithelial cells: mechanism of free radical scavenging activity. *Antioxid. Redox Signal.* 2005, 7, 32-41.

[46] Li, S.; Liu, Z.; Zhu, F.; Fan, X.; Wu, X.; Zhao, H.; Jiang, L. Curcumin lowers erlotinib resistance in non-small cell lung carcinoma cells with mutated EGF receptor. *Oncol. Res.* 2014, 21, 137-144.

[47] Yamauchi, Y.; Izumi, Y.; Yamamoto, J.; Nomori, H. Coadministration of Erlotinib and Curcumin augmentatively reduces cell viability in lung cancer cells. *Phytother. Res.* 2014, 28, 728-735.

[48] Lev-Ari, S.; Starr, A.; Katzburg, S.; Berkovich, L.; Rimmon, A.; Ben-Yosef, R.; Vexler, A.; Ron, I.; Earon, G. Curcumin induces apoptosis and inhibits growth of orthotopic human non-small cell lung cancer xenografts. *J. Nutr. Biochem.* 2014, 25, 843-850.

[49] Shishodia, S.; Potdar, P.; Gairola, C. G.; Aggarwal, B. B. Curcumin (diferuloylmethane) down-regulates cigarette smoke-induced NF-κB activation through inhibition of IκBα kinase in human lung epithelial cells: correlation with suppression of COX-2, MMP-9 and cyclin D1. *Carcinogenesis*, 2003, 24, 1269-1279.

[50] Nesbitt, J. C.; Putnam, Jr. J. B.; Walsh, G. L.; Roth, J. A.; Mountain, C. F.; Survival in early-stage non-small cell lung cancer. *Ann. Thorac. Surg.* 1995, 60, 466-472.

[51] Chen, Q.-Y.; Zheng, Y.; Jiao, D.-M.; Chen, F.-Y.; Hu, H.-Z.; Wu, Y.-Q.; Song, J.; Yan, J.; Wu, L.-J.; Lv, G.-Y. Curcumin inhibits lung cancer cell migration and invasion through Rac1-dependent signaling pathway. *J. Nutr. Biochem.* 2014, 25, 177-185.

[52] Li, Z.-C.; Zhang, L.-M.; Wang, H.-B.; Ma, J.-X.; Sun, J.-Z. Curcumin inhibits lung cancer progression and metastasis through induction of FOXO1. *Tumor Biol.* 2014, 35, 111-116.

[53] Malhotra, A.; Nair, P.; Dhawan, D. K. Study to evaluate molecular mechanics behind synergistic chemo-preventive effects of curcumin and resveratrol during lung carcinogenesis. *PloS one*, 2014, 9, e93820.

[54] Thomas, M. B.; Abbruzzese, J. L. Opportunities for targeted therapies in hepatocellular carcinoma. *J. Clin. Oncol.* 2005, 23, 8093-8108.

[55] Xu, M. X.; Zhao, L.; Deng, C.; Yang, L.; Wang, Y.; Guo, T.; Li, L.; Lin, J.; Zhang, L. Curcumin suppresses proliferation and induces apoptosis of human hepatocellular carcinoma cells via the Wnt signaling pathway. *Int. J. Oncol.* 2013, 43, 1951-1959.

[56] Kim, H. J.; Park, S. Y.; Park, O. J.; Kim, Y.-M. Curcumin suppresses migration and proliferation of Hep3B hepatocarcinoma cells through inhibition of the Wnt signaling pathway. *Mol. Med. Rep.* 2013, 8, 282-286.

[57] Wang, W.-Z.; Li, L.; Liu, M.-Y.; Jin, X.-B.; Mao, J.-W.; Pu, Q.-H.; Meng, M.-J.; Chen, X.-G.; Zhu, J.-Y. Curcumin induces FasL-related apoptosis through p38 activation in human hepatocellular carcinoma Huh7 cells. *Life Sci.* 2013, 92, 352-358.

[58] Fan, H.; Tian, W.; Ma, X. Curcumin induces apoptosis of HepG2 cells via inhibiting fatty acid synthase. *Targ. Oncol.* 2013 (DOI: 10.1007/s11523-013-0286-5), Springer-Verlag France.

[59] Jiang, J.; Jin, H.; Liu, L.; Pi, J.; Yang, F.; Cai, J. Curcumin disturbed cell-cycle distribution of HepG2 cells via cytoskeletal arrangement. *Scanning*, 2013, 35, 253-260.

[60] Dasu, M. R.; Devaraj, S.; Zhao, L.; Hwang, D. H.; Jialal, I. High glucose induces Toll-like receptor expression in human monocytes: mechanism of activation. *Diabetes*, 2008, 57, 3090-3098.

[61] Han, K.-J.; Su, X.; Xu, L.-G.; Bin, L.-H.; Zhang, J.; Shu, H.-B. Mechanisms of the TRIF-induced interferon-stimulated response element and NF-κB activation and apoptosis pathways. *J. Biol. Chem.* 2004, 279, 15652-15661.

[62] Li, P.-M.; Li, Y.-L.; Liu, B.; Wang, W.-J.; Wang, Y.-Z.; Li, Z. Curcumin inhibits MHCC97H liver cancer cells by activating ROS/TLR-4/caspase signaling pathway *Asian Pac. J. Cancer Prev.* 2014, 15, 2329-2334.

[63] Chiablaem, K.; Lirdprapamongkol, K.; Keeratichamroen, S.; Surarit, R.; Svasti, J. Curcumin suppresses vasculogenic mimicry capacity of hepatocellular carcinoma cells through STAT3 and PI3K/AKT inhibition. *Anticancer Res.* 2014, 34, 1857-1864.

[64] Lu, D.; Wang, P.; Yang, Z.; Lin, T.; Tang, L.; Li, Y.; Wo, X. Effects of curcumin on proteome of HepG2 cell. *Med. Plant*, 2013, 4, 59-63.

[65] Bae, M.-K.; Kim, S.-H.; Jeong, J.-W.; Lee, Y. M.; Kim, H.-S.; Kim, S.-R.; Yun, I.; Bae, S.-K.; Kim, K.-W. Curcumin inhibits hypoxia-induced angiogenesis via down-regulation of HIF-1. *Oncol. Rep.* 2006, 15, 1557-1562.

[66] Choi, H.; Chun, Y.-S.; Kim, S.-W.; Kim, M.-S.; Park, J.-W. Curcumin inhibits hypoxia-inducible factor-1 by degrading aryl hydrocarbon receptor nuclear translocator: a mechanism of tumor growth inhibition. *Mol. Pharmacol.* 2006, 70, 1664-1671.

[67] Kozuki, Y.; Miura, Y.; Yagasaki, K. Inhibitory effect of curcumin on the invasion of rat ascites hepatoma cells in vitro and ex vivo. *Cytotechnology*, 2001, 35, 57-63.

[68] Shan, X.; Li, Y.; Meng, X.; Wang, P.; Jiang, P.; Feng, Q. Curcumin and (-)-epigallocatechin-3-gallate attenuate acrylamide-induced proliferation in HepG2 cells. *Food Chem. Toxicol.* 2014, 66, 194-202.

[69] Nasr, M.; Selima, E.; Hamed, O.; Kazem, A. Targeting different angiogenic pathways with combination of curcumin, leflunomide and perindopril inhibits diethylnitrosamine-induced hepatocellular carcinoma in mice. *Eur. J. Pharmacol.* 2014, 723, 267-275.

[70] Shen, F.; Cai, W.-S.; Li, J.-L.; Feng, Z.; Xiao, H.-Q.; Cao, J.; Xu, B.; Liu, Q.-C. Synergism from the combination of ulinastatin and curcumin offers greater inhibition against colorectal cancer liver metastases via modulating matrix metalloproteinase-9 and E-cadherin expression. *Onco Targets Ther.* 2014, 7, 305-314.

[71] Kang, O. H.; Kim, S. B.; Seo, Y. S.; Joung, D. K.; Mun, S. H.; Choi, J. G.; Lee, Y. M.; Kang, D. G.; Lee, H. S.; Kwon, D. Y. Curcumin decreases oleic acid-induced lipid accumulation via AMPK phosphorylation in hepatocarcinoma cells. *Eur. Rev. Med. Pharmacol. Sci.* 2013, 17, 2578-2586.

[72] Shoji, M.; Nakagawa, K.; Watanabe, A.; Tsuduki, T.; Yamada, T.; Kuwahara, S.; Kimura, F.; Miyazawa, T. Comparison of the effects of curcumin and curcumin

glucuronide in human hepatocellular carcinoma HepG2 cells. *Food Chem.* 2014, 151, 126-132.

[73] Cai, X. Z.; Huang, W. Y.; Qiao, Y.; Du, S. Y.; Chen, Y.; Chen, D.; Yu, S.; Che, R. C.; Liu, N.; Jiang, Y. Inhibitory effects of curcumin on gastric cancer cells: A proteomic study of molecular targets. *Phytomedicine*, 2013, 20, 495-505.

[74] Chen, B.; Li, X.; Liu, J.; Wang, S.; Feng, W.; Lu, G.; Han, X. Inhibitory effects of curcumin on mouse stomach neoplasia and human carcinoma cell line. *Special Publication - Royal Society of Chemistry (2000), 255(Dietary Anticarcinogens and Antimutagens),* 372-375.

[75] Yu, L.-L.; Wu, J.-G.; Dai, N.; Yu, H.-G.; Si, J.-M. Curcumin reverses chemoresistance of human gastric cancer cells by downregulating the NF-κB transcription factor. *Oncol. Rep.* 2011, 26, 1197-1203.

[76] Cao, A.; Li, Q.; Yin, P.; Dong, Y.; Shi, H.; Wang, L.; Ji, G.; Xie, J.; Wu, D. Curcumin induces apoptosis in human gastric carcinoma AGS cells and colon carcinoma HT-29 cells through mitochondrial dysfunction and endoplasmic reticulum stress. *Apoptosis,* 2013, 18, 1391-1402.

[77] Koo, J. Y.; Kim, H. J.; Jung, K.-O.; Park, K.-Y. Curcumin inhibits the growth of AGS human gastric carcinoma cells in vitro and shows synergism with 5-fluorouracil. *J. Med. Food*, 2004, 7, 117-121.

[78] Lehne, G. P-glycoprotein as a drug target in the treatment of multidrug resistant cancer. *Curr. Drug Targets* 2000, 1, 85-99.

[79] Hamilton, K. O.; Topp, E.; Makagiansar, I.; Siahaan, T.; Yazdanian, M.; Audus, K. L. Multidrug resistance-associated protein-1 functional activity in Calu-3 cells. *J. Pharmacol. Exp. Ther.* 2001, 298, 1199-1205.

[80] http://www.who.int/medicines/publications/essentialmedicines/18th_EML_Final_web_ 8Jul13.pdf (Accessed date: July 26, 2014).

[81] Tang, X.-Q.; Bi, H.; Feng, J.-Q.; Cao, J.-G. Effect of curcumin on multidrug resistance in resistant human gastric carcinama cell line SGC7901/VCR. *Acta Pharmacol. Sin.* 2005, 26, 1009-1016.

[82] Johnstone, R. W.; Cretney, E.; Smyth, M. J. P-glycoprotein protects leukemia cells against caspase-dependent, but not caspase independent, cell death. *Blood*, 1999, 93, 1075-1085.

[83] Smyth, M. J.; Krasovskis, E.; Sutton, V. R.; Johnstone, R. W. The drug efflux protein, P-glycoprotein, additionally protects drug-resistant tumor cells from multiple forms of caspase-dependent apoptosis. *Proc. Natl. Acad. Sci. US,* 1998, 95, 7024-7029.

[84] Sintara, K.; Thong-Ngam, D.; Patumraj, S.; Klaikeaw, N. Curcumin attenuates gastric cancer induced by *N*-methyl-N-nitrosourea and saturated sodium chloride in rats. *J. Biomed. Biotechnol.* 2012, Article ID: 915380, 8 pp.

[85] Cheng, A.-L.; Hsu, C.-H.; Lin, J.-K.; Hsu, M.-M.; Ho, Y.-F.; Shen, T.-S.; Ko, J.-Y.; Lin, J.-T.; Lin, B.-R.; Wu, M.-S., et al. Phase I clinical trial of curcumin, a chemopreventive agent, in patients with high-risk or pre-malignant lesions. *Anticancer Res.* 2001, 21, 2895-2900.

[86] Kim, T.-D.; Berry, W. L.; Fuchs, J. R.; Schwartz, E.; Abdelhamid, D.; Etter, J.; Li, C.; Li, P.-K.; Ihnat, M. A.; Janknecht, R. Pro-growth role of the JMJD2C histone demethylase in HCT-116 colon cancer cells and identification of curcuminoids as JMJD2 inhibitors. *Am. J. Transl. Res.* 2014, 6, 236-247.

[87] Collett, G. P.; Campbell, F. C. Curcumin induces c-jun N-terminal kinase-dependent apoptosis in HCT116 human colon cancer cells. *Carcinogenesis*, 2004, 25, 2183-2189.

[88] Collett, G. P.; Campbell, F. C. Overexpression of p65/RelA potentiates curcumin-induced apoptosis in HCT116 human colon cancer cells. *Carcinogenesis*, 2006, 27, 1285-1291.

[89] Wang, X.; Wang, Q.; Ives, K. L.; Evers, B. M. Curcumin inhibits neurotensin-mediated interleukin-8 production and migration of HCT116 human colon cancer cells. *Clin. Cancer Res.* 2006, 12, 5346-5355.

[90] Kujundzic, R. N.; Grbesa, I.; Ivkic, M.; Katdare, M.; Gall-Troselj, K. Curcumin downregulates H19 gene transcription in tumor cells. *J. Cell Biochem.* 2008, 104, 1781-1792.

[91] Milacic, V.; Banerjee, S.; Landis-Piwowar, K. R.; Sarkar, F. H.; Majumdar, A. P. N.; Dou, Q. P. curcumin inhibits the proteasome activity in human colon cancer cells *in vitro* and *in vivo*. *Cancer Res.* 2008, 68, 7283-7292.

[92] Feinberg, A. P.; Ohlsson, R.; Henikoff, S. The epigenetic progenitor origin of human cancer. *Nat. Rev. Genet.* 2006, 7, 21-33.

[93] Wong, J. J.; Hawkins, N. J.; Ward, R. L. Colorectal cancer: a model for epigenetic tumorigenesis. *Gut*, 2007, 56, 140-148.

[94] Link, A.; Balaguer, F.; Shen, Y.; Lozano, J. J.; Leung, H.-C. E.; Boland, C. R.; Goel, A. Curcumin modulates DNA methylation in colorectal cancer cells. *PLoS One*, 2013, 8, e57709.

[95] Patel, A. S.; Lin, L.; Geyer, A.; Haspel, J. A.; An, C. H.; Cao, J.; Rosas, I. O.; Morse, D. Autophagy in idiopathic pulmonary fibrosis. *PLoS One*, 2012, 7, e41394.

[96] Lin, N.-Y.; Beyer, C.; Giessl, A.; Kireva, T.; Scholtysek, C.; Uderhardt, S.; Munoz, L. E.; Dees, C.; Distler, A.; Wirtz, S.; Kroenke, G.; Spencer, B.; Distler, O.; Schett, G.; Distler, J. H. W. Autophagy regulates TNFα-mediated joint destruction in experimental arthritis. *Ann. Rheum. Dis.* 2013, 72, 761-768.

[97] Mosieniak, G.; Adamowicz, M.; Alster, O.; Jaskowiak, H.; Szczepankiewicz, A. A.; Wilczynski, G. M; Ciechomska, I. A.; Sikora, E. Curcumin induces permanent growth arrest of human colon cancer cells: link between senescence and autophagy. *Mech. Ageing Dev.* 2012, 133, 444-455.

[98] Kantara, C.; O'Connell, M.; Sarkar, S.; Moya, S.; Ullrich, R.; Singh, P. Curcumin promotes autophagic survival of a subset of colon cancer stem cells, which are ablated by DCLK1-siRNA. *Cancer Res.* 2014, 74, 2487-2498.

[99] Wu, H.; Reynolds, A. B.; Kanner, S. B.; Vines, R. R.; Parsons, J. T. Identification and characterization of a novel cytoskeleton-associated pp60src substrate. *Mol. Cell. Biol.* 1991, 11, 5113-5124.

[100] Radhakrishnan, V. M.; Kojs, P.; Young, G.; Ramalingam, R.; Bhumasamudram, J.; Mash, E. A.; Martinez, J. D.; Ghishan, F. K.; Kiela, P. R. pTyr421 cortactin is overexpressed in colon cancer and is dephosphorylated by curcumin involvement of non-receptor type 1 protein tyrosine phosphatase (PTPN1). *PLoS One*, 2014, 9, e 85796/1-e85796/13, 13 pp.

[101] Han, X.; Xu, B.; Beevers, C. S.; Odaka, Y.; Chen, L.; Liu, L.; Luo, Y.; Zhou, H.; Chen, W.; Shen, T.; Huang, S. Curcumin inhibits protein phosphatases 2A and 5, leading to activation of mitogen-activated protein kinases and death in tumor cells. *Carcinogenesis*, 2012, 33, 868-875.

[102] Watson, J. L.; Hill, R.; Yaffe, P. B.; Greenshields, A.; Walsh, M.; Lee, P. W.; Giacomantonio, C. A.; Hoskin, D. W. Curcumin causes superoxide anion production and p53-independent apoptosis in human colon cancer cells. *Cancer Lett.* 2010, 297, 1-8.

[103] Shehzad, A.; Lee, J.; Huh, T.-L.; Lee, Y. S. Curcumin induces apoptosis in human colorectal carcinoma (HCT-15) cells by regulating expression of Prp4 and p53. *Mol. Cells*, 2013, 35, 526-532.

[104] Chen, A.; Xu, J.; Johnson, A. C. Curcumin inhibits human colon cancer cell growth by suppressing gene expression of epidermal growth factor receptor through reducing the activity of the transcription factor Egr-1. *Oncogene*, 2006, 25, 278-287.

[105] Su, C.-C.; Lin, J.-G.; Li, T.-M.; Chung, J.-G.; Yang, J.-S.; Ip, S.-W.; Lin, W.-C.; Chen, G.-W. Curcumin-induced apoptosis of human colon cancer colo 205 cells through the production of ROS Ca2+ and the activation of caspase-3. *Anticancer Res.* 2006, 26, 4379-4390.

[106] Chen, J.-C.; Hwang, J.-M.; Chen, G.-W.; Tsou, M.-F.; Hsia, T.-C.; Chung, J.-G. Curcumin decreases the DNA adduct formation, arylamines *N*-acetyltransferase activity and gene expression in human colon tumor cells (colo 205). *In Vivo*, 2003, 17, 301-309.

[107] Shakibaei, M.; Buhrmann, C.; Kraehe, P.; Shayan, P.; Lueders, C.; Goel, A. Curcumin chemosensitizes 5-Fluorouracil resistant MMR-deficient human colon cancer cells in high density cultures. *PLoS One*, 2014, 9, e85397/1-e85397/12, 12 pp.

[108] Sandur, S. K.; Deorukhkar, A.; Pandey, M. K.; Pabon, A. M.; Shentu, S.; Guha, S.; Aggarwal, B. B.; Krishnan, S. *Int. J. Radiat. Oncol. Biol. Phys.* 2009, 75, 534-542.

[109] Du, B.; Jiang, L.; Xia, Q.; Zhong, L. Synergistic inhibitory effects of curcumin and 5-fluorouracil on the growth of the human colon cancer cell line HT-29. *Chemotherapy*, 2006, 52, 23-28.

[110] Shakibaei, M.; Mobasheri, A.; Lueders, C.; Busch, F.; Shayan, P.; Goel, A. Curcumin enhances the effect of chemotherapy against colorectal cancer cells by inhibition of NF-κB and Src protein kinase signaling pathways. *PLoS One*, 2013, 8, e57218.

[111] Ataee, R.; Oufkir, T.; Ataee, A.; Vaillancourt, C. The serotonin 5-HT2A receptor antagonist ritanserin induces apoptosis in human colorectal cancer and acts in synergy with curcumin. Edited By: Zarzuela, A.; Jimenez, R. In: *European Congress of Pharmacology*, 6th, Granada, Spain, July 17-20, 2012 (2013), 105-110, 6 pp.

[112] Nautiyal, J.; Kanwar, S. S.; Yu, Y.; Majumdar, A. P. N. Combination of dasatinib and curcumin eliminates chemo-resistant colon cancer cells. *J. Mol. Signal.* 2011, 6, 7.

[113] Nautiyal, J.; Banerjee, S.; Kanwar, S. S; Yu, Y.; Patel, B. B.; Sarkar, F. H.; Majumdar, A. P. N. Curcumin enhances dasatinib-induced inhibition of growth and transformation of colon cancer cells. *Int. J. Cancer*, 2011, 128, 951-961.

[114] Majumdar, A. P. N.; Banerjee, S.; Nautiyal, J.; Patel, B. B.; Patel, V.; Du, J.; Yu, Y.; Elliott, A. A.; Levi, E.; Sarkar, F. H. Curcumin synergizes with resveratrol to inhibit colon cancer. *Nutr. Cancer*, 2009, 61, 544-553.

[115] Lev-Ari, S.; Strier, L.; Kazanov, D.; Madar-Shapiro, L.; Dvory-Sobol, H.; Pinchuk, I.; Marian, B.; Lichtenberg, D.; Arber, N. Celecoxib and curcumin synergistically inhibit the growth of colorectal cancer cells. *Clin. Cancer Res.* 2005, 11, 6738-6744.

[116] Sharma, R. A.; Euden, S. A.; Platton, S. L.; Cooke, D. N.; Shafayat, A.; Hewitt, H. R.; Marczylo, T. H.; Morgan, B.; Hemingway, D.; Plummer, S. M.; Pirmohamed, M.;

Gescher, A. J.; Steward, W. P. Phase I clinical trial of oral curcumin: Biomarkers of systemic activity and compliance. *Clin. Cancer Res.* 2004, 10, 6847-6854.

[117] Irving, G. R. B.; Howells, L. M.; Sale, S.; Kralj-Hans, I.; Atkin, W. S.; Clark, S. K.; Britton, R. G.; Jones, D. J. L.; Scott, E. N.; Berry, D. P.; Hemingway, D.; Miller, A. S.; Brown, K.; Gescher, A. J.; Steward, W. P. Prolonged biologically active colonic tissue levels of curcumin achieved after oral administration-A clinical pilot study including assessment of patient acceptability. *Cancer Prev. Res.* 2013, 6, 119-128.

[118] Hua, W.-F.; Fu, Y.-S.; Liao, Y.-J.; Xia, W.-J.; Chen, Y.-C.; Zeng, Y.-X.; Kung, H.-F.; Xie, D. Curcumin induces down-regulation of EZH2 expression through the MAPK pathway in MDA-MB-435 human breast cancer cells. *Eur. J. Pharmacol.* 2010, 637, 16-21.

[119] Hendrayani, S.-F.; Al-Khalaf, H. H.; Aboussekhra, A. Curcumin triggers p16-dependent senescence in active breast cancer-associated fibroblasts and suppresses their paracrine procarcinogenic effects. *Neoplasia*, 2013, 15, 631-640.

[120] Ruijter, T. C.; Veeck, J.; Hoon, J. P. J.; Engeland, M.; Tjan-Heijnen, V. C. Characteristics of triple-negative breast cancer. *J. Cancer Res. Clin. Oncol.* 2011, 137, 183-192.

[121] Siziopikou, K. P.; Ariga, R.; Proussaloglou, K. E.; Gattuso, P.; Cobleigh, M. The challenging estrogen receptor-negative/progesterone receptor-negative/HER-2-negative patient: a promising candidate for epidermal growth factor receptor-targeted therapy? *Breast J.* 2006, 12, 360-362.

[122] Sun, X.-D.; Liu, X.-E.; Huang, D.-S. Curcumin induces apoptosis of triple-negative breast cancer cells by inhibition of EGFR expression. *Mol. Med. Rep.* 2012, 6, 1267-1270.

[123] Rowe, D. L.; Ozbay, T.; O'Regan, R. M.; Nahta, R. Modulation of the BRCA1 protein and induction of apoptosis in triple negative breast cancer cell lines by the polyphenolic compound curcumin. *Breast Cancer: Basic Clin. Res.* 2009, 3, 61-75.

[124] Quiroga, A.; Quiroga, P. L.; Martinez, E.; Soria, E. A.; Valentich, M. A. Anti-breast cancer activity of curcumin on the human oxidation-resistant cells ZR-75-1 with γ-glutamyltranspeptidase inhibition. *J. Exp. Ther. Oncol.* 2010, 8, 261-266.

[125] Liu, Q.; Loo, W. T. Y.; Sze, S. C. W.; Tong, Y. Curcumin inhibits cell proliferation of MDA-MB-231 and BT-483 breast cancer cells mediated by down-regulation of NFκB, cyclinD and MMP-1 transcription. *Phytomedicine*, 2009, 16, 916-922.

[126] Long, L.; Cao, Y.-D. Down-regulation of Notch1 and Nf-κB by curcumin in breast cancer cells MDA-MB-231. *Chin. J. Cancer Res.* 2008, 20, 294-300.

[127] Choudhuri, T.; Pal, S.; Agwarwal, M. L.; Das, T.; Sa, G. Curcumin induces apoptosis in human breast cancer cells through p53-dependent Bax induction. *FEBS Lett.* 2002, 512, 334-340.

[128] Mitri, Z.; Constantine, T.; O'Regan, R. The HER2 receptor in breast cancer: pathophysiology, clinical use, and new advances in therapy. *Chemother. Res. Pract.* 2012, Article ID: 743193, 7 pp.

[129] Lai, H.-W.; Chien, S.-Y.; Kuo, S.-J.; Tseng, L.-M.; Lin, H.-Y.; Chi, C.-W.; Chen, D.-R. The potential utility of curcumin in the treatment of HER-2-overexpressed breast cancer: an *in vitro* and *in vivo* comparison study with Herceptin. *Evid. Based Complement. Alternat. Med.* eCAM (2012), Article ID: 2012486568.

[130] Gupta, G. P.; Massagué, J. Cancer metastasis: building a framework. *Cell*, 2006, 127, 679-695.

[131] Charpentier, M. S.; Whipple, R. A.; Vitolo, M. I.; Boggs, A. E.; Slovic, J.; Thompson, K.N.; Bhandary, L.; Martin, S.S. Curcumin targets breast cancer stem-like cells with microtentacles that persist in mammospheres and promote reattachment. *Cancer Res.* 2014, 74, 1250-1260.

[132] Kronski, E.; Fiori, M. E.; Barbieri, O.; Astigiano, S.; Mirisola, V.; Killian, P. H.; Bruno, A.; Pagani, A.; Rovera, F.; Pfeffer, U.; Sommerhoff, C. P.; Noonan, D. M.; Nerlich, A. G.; Fontana, L.; Bachmeier, B. E. miR181b is induced by the chemopreventive polyphenol curcumin and inhibits breast cancer metastasis via down-regulation of the inflammatory cytokines CXCL1 and -2. *Mol. Oncol.* 2014, 8, 581-595.

[133] Zong, H.; Wang, F.; Fan, Q.-X.; Wang, L.-X. Curcumin inhibits metastatic progression of breast cancer cell through suppression of urokinase-type plasminogen activator by NF-kappa B signaling pathways. *Mol. Biol. Rep.* 2012, 39, 4803-4808.

[134] Kim, J.-M.; Noh, E.-M.; Kwon, K.-B.; Kim, J.-S.; You, Y.-O.; Hwang, J.-K.; Hwang, B.-M.; Kim, B.-S.; Lee, S.-H.; Lee, S. J.; Jung, S. H.; Youn, H. J.; Lee, Y.-R. Curcumin suppresses the TPA-induced invasion through inhibition of PKCα-dependent MMP-expression in MCF-7 human breast cancer cells. *Phytomedicine*, 2012, 19, 1085-1092.

[135] Kim, S.-R.; Park, H.-J.; Bae, Y.-H.; Ahn, S.-C.; Wee, H.-J.; Yun, I.; Jang, H.-O.; Bae, M.-K.; Bae, S.-K. Curcumin down-regulates visfatin expression and inhibits breast cancer cell invasion. *Endocrinology*, 2012, 153, 554-563.

[136] Chiu, T.-L.; Su, C.-C. Curcumin inhibits proliferation and migration by increasing the Bax to Bcl-2 ratio and decreasing NF-κBp65 expression in breast cancer MDA-MB-231 cells. *Int. J. Mol. Med.* 2009, 23, 469-475.

[137] Kim, H. I.; Huang, H.; Cheepala, S.; Huang, S.; Chung, J. Curcumin inhibition of integrin (α6β4)-dependent breast cancer cell motility and invasion. *Cancer Prev. Res.* 2008, 1, 385-391.

[138] Prasad, C. P.; Rath, G.; Mathur, S.; Bhatnagar, D.; Ralhan, R. Expression analysis of maspin in invasive ductal carcinoma of breast and modulation of its expression by curcumin in breast cancer cell lines. *Chem. Biol. Interact.* 2010, 183, 455-461.

[139] Kim, M.-S.; Kang, H.-J.; Moon, A. Inhibition of invasion and induction of apoptosis by curcumin in H-ras-transformed MCF10A human breast epithelial cells. *Arch. Pharmacal Res.* 2001, 24, 349-354.

[140] Kizhakkayil, J.; Thayyullathil, F.; Chathoth, S.; Hago, A.; Patel, M.; Galadari, S. Modulation of curcumin-induced Akt phosphorylation and apoptosis by PI3K inhibitor in MCF-7 cells. *Biochem. Biophys. Res. Commun.* 2010, 394, 476-481.

[141] Chen, W.-C.; Lai, Y.-A.; Lin, Y.-C.; Ma, J.-W.; Huang, L.-F.; Yang, N.-S.; Ho, C.-T.; Kuo, S.-C.; Way, T.-D. Curcumin suppresses doxorubicin-induced epithelial-mesenchymal transition via the inhibition of TGF-β and PI3K/AKT signaling pathways in triple-negative breast cancer cells. *J. Agric. Food Chem.* 2013, 61, 11817-11824.

[142] Zhou, Q.-M.; Zhang, H.; Lu, Y.-Y.; Wang, X.-F.; Su, S.-B. Curcumin reduced the side effects of mitomycin C by inhibiting GRP58-mediated DNA cross-linking in MCF-7 breast cancer xenografts. *Cancer Sci.* 2009, 100, 2040-2045.

[143] Kang, H. J.; Lee, S. H.; Price, J. E.; Kim, L. S. Curcumin suppresses the paclitaxel-induced nuclear factor-κB in breast cancer cells and potentiates the growth inhibitory effect of paclitaxel in a breast cancer nude mice model. *Breast J.* 2009, 15, 223-229.

[144] Cheah, Y. H.; Nordin, F. J.; Sarip, R.; Tee, T. T.; Azimahtol, H. L. P.; Sirat, H. M.; Rashid, B. A.; Abdullah, N. R.; Abd Ismail, Z. Combined xanthorrhizol- curcumin exhibits synergistic growth inhibitory activity via apoptosis induction in human breast cancer cells MDA-MB-231. *Cancer Cell Int.* 2009, 9.

[145] Lin, Y.-C.; Chen, H.-W.; Kuo, Y.-C.; Chang, Y.-F.; Lee, Y.-J.; Hwang, J.-J. Therapeutic efficacy evaluation of curcumin on human oral squamous cell carcinoma xenograft using multimodalities of molecular imaging. *Am. J. Chin. Med.* 2010, 38, 343-358.

[146] Lin, Y.-T.; Wang, L.-F.; Hsu, Y.-C. Curcuminoids suppress the growth of pharynx and nasopharyngeal carcinoma cells through induced apoptosis. *J. Agric. Food Chem.* 2009, 57, 3765-3770.

[147] Koon, H. K.; Leung, A. W. N.; Yue, K. K. M.; Mak, N. K. Photodynamic effect of curcumin on NPC/CNE2 cells. *J. Environ. Pathol. Toxicol. Oncol.* 2006, 25, 205-215.

[148] Xie, Y.-Q.; Wu, X.-B.; Tang, S.-Q. Curcumin treatment alters ERK-1/2 signaling in vitro and inhibits nasopharyngeal carcinoma proliferation in mouse xenografts. *Int. J. Clin. Exp. Med.* 2014, 7, 108-114.

[149] O'Sullivan-Coyne, G.; O'Sullivan, G. C.; O'Donovan, T. R.; Piwocka, K.; McKenna, S.L. Curcumin induces apoptosis-independent death in oesophageal cancer cells. *Br. J. Cancer*, 2009, 101, 1585-1595.

[150] Subramaniam, D.; Ponnurangam, S.; Ramamoorthy, P.; Standing, D.; Battafarano, R. J.; Anant, S.; Sharma, P. Curcumin induces cell death in esophageal cancer cells through modulating Notch signaling. *PLoS One*, 2012, 7, e30590.

[151] Liu, T.-Y.; Tan, Z.-J.; Jiang, L.; Gu, J.-F.; Wu, X.-S.; Cao, Y.; Li, M.-L.; Wu, K.-J.; Liu, Y.-B. Curcumin induces apoptosis in gallbladder carcinoma cell line GBC-SD cells. *Cancer Cell Int.* 2013, 13, 64.

[152] Ono, M.; Higuchi, T.; Takeshima, M.; Chen, C.; Nakano, S. Antiproliferative and apoptosis-inducing activity of curcumin against human gallbladder adenocarcinoma cells. *Anticancer Res.* 2013, 33, 1861-1866.

[153] Bimonte, S.; Barbieri, A.; Palma, G.; Luciano, A.; Rea, D.; Arra, C. Curcumin inhibits tumor growth and angiogenesis in an orthotopic mouse model of human pancreatic cancer. *BioMed Res. Int.* 2013, 2013810423.

[154] Youns, M.; Fathy, G. M. Upregulation of extrinsic apoptotic pathway in curcumin-mediated antiproliferative effect on human pancreatic carcinogenesis. *J. Cell. Biochem.* 2013, 114, 2654-2665.

[155] Mitra, A.; Chakrabarti, J.; Banerji, A.; Chatterjee, A.; Das, B. R. Curcumin, a potential inhibitor of MMP-2 in human laryngeal squamous carcinoma cells HEp2. *J. Environ. Pathol. Toxicol. Oncol.* 2006, 25, 679-689.

[156] Anuchapreeda, S.; Leechanachai, P.; Smith, M. M.; Ambudkar, S. V.; Limtrakul, P. Modulation of P-glycoprotein expression and function by curcumin in multidrug-resistant human KB cells. *Biochem. Pharmacol.* 2002, 64, 573-582.

[157] Prusty, B. K.; Das, B. C. Constitutive activation of transcription factor AP-1 in cervical cancer and suppression of human papillomavirus (HPV) transcription and AP-1 activity in HeLa cells by curcumin. *Int. J. Cancer*, 2005, 113, 951-960.

[158] Watson, J. L.; Greenshields, A.; Hill, R.; Hilchie, A.; Lee, P. W.; Giacomantonio, C. A.; Hoskin, D. W. Curcumin-induced apoptosis in ovarian cancinoma cells is p53-independent and involves p38 mitogen-activated protein kinase activation and

downregulation of Bcl-2 and survivin expression and Akt signaling. *Mol. Carcinog.* 2010, 49, 13-24.

[159] Saydmohammed, M.; Joseph, D.; Syed, V. Curcumin suppresses constitutive activation of STAT-3 by up-regulating protein inhibitor of activated STAT-3 (PIAS-3) in ovarian and endometrial cancer cells. *J. Cell. Biochem.* 2010, 110, 447-456.

[160] Srivastava, R. K.; Chen, Q.; Siddiqui, I.; Sarva, K.; Shankar, S. Linkage of curcumin-induced cell cycle arrest and apoptosis by cyclin-dependent kinase inhibitor p21/WAF1/CIP1. *Cell Cycle*, 2007, 6, 2953-2961.

[161] Deeb, D.; Jiang, H.; Gao, X.; Al-Holou, S.; Danyluk, A. L.; Dulchavsky, S. A.; Gautam, S. C. Curcumin [1,7-bis(4-hydroxy-3-methoxyphenyl)-1-6-heptadine-3,5-dione; C21H20O6] sensitizes human prostate cancer cells to tumor necrosis factor-related apoptosis-inducing ligand/Apo2L-induced apoptosis by suppressing nuclear factor-κB via inhibition of the prosurvival Akt signaling pathway. *J. Pharm. Exp. Ther.* 2007, 321, 616-625.

[162] Zhou, C.; Zhao, X.-M.; Li, X.-F.; Wang, C.; Zhang, X.-T.; Liu, X.-Z.; Ding, X.-F.; Xiang, S.-L.; Zhang, J. Curcumin inhibits AP-2γ-induced apoptosis in the human malignant testicular germ cells in vitro. *Acta Pharmacol. Sin.* 2013, 34, 1192-1200.

[163] Seo, B. R.; Min, K.-J.; Kwon, T. K.; Cho, I. J.; Kim, S. C. Curcumin significantly enhances dual PI3K/Akt and mTOR inhibitor NVP-BEZ235-induced apoptosis in human renal carcinoma Caki cells through down-regulation of p53-dependent Bcl-2 expression and inhibition of Mcl-1 protein stability. *PloS One*, 2014, 9, e95588.

[164] Li, G.; Chong, T.; Wang, Z. Curcumin induces the expression of NF-κB and Bcl-2/Bax in human renal cell carcinoma cell line ACHN. *JNMU*, 2009, 23, 386-391.

[165] Du, W.-Z.; Feng, Y.; Wang, X.-F.; Piao, X.-Y.; Cui, Y.-Q.; Chen, L.-C.; Lei, X.-H.; Sun, X.; Liu, X.; Wang, H.-B.; Li, X.-F.; Yang, D.-B.; Sun, Y.; Zhao, Z.-F.; Jiang, T.; Li, Y.-L.; Jiang, C.-L. Curcumin suppresses malignant glioma cells growth and induces apoptosis by inhibition of SHH/GLI1 signaling pathway *in vitro* and *vivo*. *CNS Neurosci. Ther.* 2013, 19, 926-936.

[166] Xu, X.; Qin, J.; Liu, W. Curcumin inhibits the invasion of thyroid cancer cells via down-regulation of PI3K/Akt signaling pathway. *Gene*, 2014, 546, 226-232.

[167] Zhang, C.-Y.; Zhang, L.; Yu, H.-X.; Bao, J.-D.; Lu, R.-R. Curcumin inhibits the metastasis of K1 papillary thyroid cancer cells via modulating E-cadherin and matrix metalloproteinase-9 expression. *Biotechnol. Lett.* 2013, 35, 995-1000.

[168] Bharti, A. C.; Donato, N.; Aggarwal, B. B. Curcumin (diferuloylmethane) inhibits constitutive and IL-6-inducible STAT3 phosphorylation in human multiple myeloma cells. *J. Immunol.* 2003, 171, 3863-3871.

[169] Bharti, A. C.; Donato, N.; Singh, S.; Aggarwal, B. B. Curcumin(diferuloylmethane) down-regulates the constitutive activation of nuclear factor-κB and IκBα kinase in human multiple myeloma cells, leading to suppression of proliferation and induction of apoptosis. *Blood*, 2003, 101, 1053-1062.

[170] Guo, Y.; Shan, Q.; Gong, Y.; Lin, J.; Shi, F.; Shi, R.; Yang, X. Curcumin induces apoptosis via simultaneously targeting AKT/mTOR and RAF/MEK/ERK survival signaling pathways in human leukemia THP-1 cells. *Pharmazie*, 2014, 69, 229-233.

[171] Gopal, P. K.; Paul, M.; Paul, S. Curcumin induces caspase mediated apoptosis in JURKAT cells by disrupting the redox balance. *Asian Pac. J. Cancer Prev.: APJCP*, 2014, 15, 93-100.

[172] Bandyopadhyay, D.; Banik, B. K. Bismuth nitrate-induced microwave-assisted expeditious synthesis of vanillin from curcumin. *Org. Med. Chem. Lett.* 2012, 2, 15, 4 pp.

[173] Goel, A.; Aggarwal, B. B. Curcumin, the golden spice from Indian saffron, is a chemosensitizer and radiosensitizer for tumors and chemoprotector and radioprotector for normal organs. *Nutr. Cancer*, 2010, 62, 919-930.

In: Horizons in Cancer Research. Volume 55
Editor: Hiroto S. Watanabe

ISBN: 978-1-63463-228-7
© 2015 Nova Science Publishers, Inc.

Chapter 2

Diagnosis of Thyroid Cancers in the Era of Molecular Medicine: New Paradigm in Cytologic and Histologic Diagnosis of Thyroid Cancer?

Lewis A. Hassell[1,], Ericka Olgaard[2]*
and S. Terence Dunn[3]

[1]University of Oklahoma Health Sciences Center; Anatomic Pathology;
Department of Pathology; Oklahoma City, OK, US
[2]University of Oklahoma Health Sciences Center; Department of Pathology;
Oklahoma City, OK, US
[3]University of Oklahoma Health Sciences Center; Molecular Pathology Laboratory;
Department of Pathology; Oklahoma City, OK, US

Abstract

Background: The Bethesda system for standardized reporting of thyroid fine needle aspiration (FNA) cytology has positively impacted clarity of communication of results and management of patients evaluated for thyroid nodules. Problematic areas still exist in the triage of some of these samples, particularly those in the categories of "follicular lesion with atypia of uncertain significance" and "follicular lesion".

The discovery of a variety of molecular markers associated with various thyroid neoplasms offers both opportunity and challenges in appropriate application to the patient with a thyroid nodule. Additionally, a transition from molecular marker to therapeutic target begins to change the treatment paradigm both before and following surgical intervention.

Methods: The literature on molecular and genetic abnormalities in thyroid lesions is reviewed. Potentially useful markers for distinguishing currently problematic categories

* Tel: (405) 271-4062; E-mail: lewis-hassell@ouhsc.edu.

of FNA cytologic samples, especially non-diagnostic samples, atypia of uncertain significance, and follicular lesions are discussed. The predictive value of molecular analyses in these settings is examined. The role of molecular evaluation of resected tumors is also reviewed.

Results: Evaluation of FNA samples with negative or suboptimal follicular cytology for Ras gene mutations may be useful in detecting potentially significant follicular lesions (carcinomas) but is quite low in overall yield. Cytologic samples with atypia of uncertain significance, as well as those classified as follicular lesions or suspicious for malignancy, which may include the possibility of papillary carcinomas, may be fruitfully evaluated using a panel of molecular tests for *BRAF, RET*/PTC, *PAX8/PPARγ1* and Ras genes. Other emerging markers have potential utility in the work-up of thyroid lesions.

Introduction and Background

Thyroid cancer is the most common endocrine malignancy. Overall, however, thyroid cancer is quite rare, constituting less than 1.5% of all cancers in adults and 3% of all cancers in children. In 2012, it is estimated that approximately 56,500 cases of thyroid cancer (13,250 men and 43,210 women) will be diagnosed in the United States alone. However, the prognosis associated with thyroid cancer is generally favorable and fewer than 1,800 will die per year from thyroid cancer in the USA, representing less than 0.5% of all cancer deaths [1].

While the majority of thyroid cancer is papillary (approx 75%), the greatest mortality is associated with follicular cancer, where the cause-specific mortality rate is approximately 30% at 20 years [2]. Despite the increased frequency of new cases of thyroid cancer in recent decades in the USA (6.6% annual change between 1997-2009), presumably due to increased detection of small papillary carcinomas, mortality rates as a consequence of thyroid cancers have not shifted significantly over time. Worldwide frequencies for thyroid cancer likely approximate estimates for the USA.

The majority of thyroid cancers are sporadic (non-familial), well-differentiated and arise from the follicular epithelial cells. Three separate subgroups with distinct clinical behaviors are recognized, papillary, follicular, and Hürthle cell. Papillary thyroid cancer (PTC) which constitutes the majority of thyroid cancers (approx. 80%), generally occurs in individuals between 30 and 50 years of age and has a 10-year survival of >90%. By contrast, follicular thyroid cancer (FTC), which occurs in slightly older individuals (>40 years of age), constitutes only 10% of thyroid cancers but has the greatest associated mortality; 10-year survival rates range from 40 to 90%, indicating significant heterogeneity within this disease entity. Hürthle cell carcinoma is the least frequent (3 to 10%) of differentiated thyroid cancers. While the World Health Organization (WHO) considers these neoplasms as a variant of FTC and describes them as follicular carcinoma, oxyphilic type, many investigators regard them as distinct neoplasms. Hürthle cells can also be observed in non-neoplastic conditions of the thyroid, such as Hashimoto thyroiditis and nodular and toxic goiter, often making this a challenging diagnosis. Hürthle cell cancer, defined as being composed of at least 75% Hürthle cells, has the highest incidence of metastasis among the differentiated thyroid cancers and behaves aggressively. Overall survival rates vary depending on the series, but are generally worse than FTC. One study showed a 40% disease-free survival at 10 years [3].

Poorly differentiated (PDTC) and anaplastic thyroid cancers (ATC) arising from the follicular epithelium, either *de novo* or from the progression of pre-existing papillary or follicular carcinomas, are the most aggressive thyroid malignancies. While they account for only 2 to 5% of all thyroid cancers, they comprise approximately 40% of all thyroid cancer deaths. The overall 5-year survival rate is reportedly less than 10% [4]. In ATC, the one-year overall survival is 16 to 19% with a median survival of only 4 months [5]. Peak incidence of PDTC and ATC occurs between 50 and 70 years of age.

Medullary thyroid carcinoma (MTC) is a neuroendocrine tumor arising from parafollicular C cells and accounts for 3 to 5% of all thyroid cancers. Sporadic forms of the disease show a peak incidence between 40 and 50 years of age and typically demonstrate a relatively indolent progression, while MTC associated with multiple endocrine neoplasia (MEN) occurs during the second or third decade of life and tends to have a more aggressive clinical course.

The classification of thyroid neoplasms has been significantly revised in the last 20 years, reflecting a deepening understanding of the histologic characteristics and clinical behaviors of these tumors, which is reinforced in many ways by the expanding knowledge of molecular events in these neoplasms. Likewise, evaluation and management of thyroid nodules has changed dramatically over the past three decades. Noteworthy diagnostic advances to the area of thyroid cancer evaluation include radionuclide scintigraphy and ultrasound (US) imaging studies. Only 5 to 10% of thyroid cancers are clinically palpable and a major challenge exists in differentiating the few clinically significant nodules from the many benign ones [6]. The introduction of radionuclide scintigraphy imaging allowed a functional classification of thyroid nodules into those taking-up or trapping tracer radionuclide ("hot") and those with decreased radiotracer activity ("cold"). Hot nodules (which are typically adenomas) are more often benign than cold lesions so this technological advance alone excluded many nodules from the need for further evaluation [7]. However, the remaining cold nodules, while containing an enriched proportion of neoplastic lesions, still included many benign entities. More recently, ultrasound (US) has become the preferred modality for initial evaluation of palpable thyroid nodules, detection of local tumor recurrence, and in searching for primary lesions in patients with metastases [5]. In some populations, it is a screening modality for thyroid disease. It is estimated that only 4 to 7% of thyroid nodules detected by US are palpable in adult patients; US can differentiate intra-thyroid cysts down to 2 mm and solid tumors as small as 3 mm [8]. Besides identifying many more non-palpable nodules, certain features of US can also help in defining the potentially benign or malignant nature of a given nodule. Such information can help guide surgical procedures and direct biopsy sampling. Other more advanced imaging modalities, such as computed tomography and magnetic resonance imaging, have limited roles in characterizing thyroid nodules but are effective in detecting regional and distant metastases.

Another major advance in the management of patients with thyroid nodules came with the popularization of percutaneous fine needle aspiration (FNA) biopsy during the last few decades of the 20th century. This relatively simple, readily available, inexpensive, and accurate technique combined with cytologic evaluation is currently the standard pre-operative tool used for assessing thyroid nodules. When malignant features are observed, the patient generally proceeds to surgery for total or near-total thyroidectomy. However, there remains a substantial group of cases in which FNA findings are non-diagnostic (i.e., insufficient cells and/or colloid) or cannot reliably distinguish malignant features from benign proliferation (i.e., indeterminate category) [9, 10]. In fact, cytological diagnosis of up to 40% of cases can remain indeterminate for malignancy [11]. The National Cancer Institute "Thyroid Fine

Needle Aspiration (FNA) State of the Science Conference" in October 2007, further defined and delineated this indeterminate category of FNAs into three subcategories, i.e., follicular lesion of undetermined significance (FLUS), follicular or oncocytic (Hürthle cell) neoplasm, and suspicious for malignancy with predicted probabilities or risk for malignancy associated with these subcategories at 5-10%, 20-30%, and 50-75%, respectively [12]. Based on the risk of malignancy data examined at this consensus conference, management recommendations are associated with each of the classifications in the proposed diagnostic categories espoused in the conference documents, collectively known as "the Bethesda system." Currently, diagnostic thyroidectomy would be recommended for patients with indeterminate lesions to exclude the possibility of malignancy. Clinical implementation of the Bethesda system for classification and management of thyroid nodules has made a positive impact on patient management [13, 14]. While palpation-guided FNA can be performed with high levels of success in many circumstances, several studies have clearly demonstrated that US-guided FNAs reduce the rates of non-diagnostic and false-negative aspirates [15, 16]. In one series, patients with initial benign results on palpation-guided FNA were re-assessed using US-guided FNA, which led to reclassification and diagnosis of 14% more cancers [17].

Despite these advances in the evaluation of thyroid nodules, there are still situations in which our best diagnostic practices yield inconclusive results. FNA of follicular lesions are notoriously problematic, for instance, because benign follicular adenomas have similar cytologic appearance to malignant FTC and a definitive diagnosis of FTC currently requires histological demonstration of capsular or vascular invasion in a resected thyroid specimen. In addition, FNA cannot accurately distinguish between benign and malignant Hürthle cell tumors. Obviously, when a patient is subjected to surgery for a lesion ultimately found to be benign, the system has not provided the best outcome. Similarly, when a patient is mistakenly assigned to a low-risk group but ultimately is found to have a malignancy, the evaluation protocols are suboptimal. There is an obvious need for more sensitive and reliable adjunct tests to complement current diagnostic methods. In recent years, the addition of molecular approaches to the evaluation of thyroid nodules has offered significant promise in reducing or resolving this conundrum, and these are already changing diagnostic algorithms for work-up of preoperative FNA biopsies on thyroid nodules. Also, various biomarkers have potential utility in defining prognosis and therapeutic regimens for thyroid cancer patients.

Moreover, the paradigm of treatment is changing as the biologic individuality of these tumors is revealed through molecular analysis, and as further targets for therapy are identified along with specific drugs to attack those targets. Clearly, this model of very personalized or individualized treatment also has significant implications for the initial evaluation of patient and tumor. The following sections detail some of the common molecular markers of the different thyroid cancers that have been revealed in the past decades and describe ways in which they may be used in defining disease, establishing treatment, and making prognostication decisions.

Papillary Thyroid Carcinoma

Papillary thyroid carcinoma accounts for the majority of thyroid malignancies, and, at least in the Western world, is increasing in frequency [1]. For instance, from 1973 to 2002, the incidence of PTC increased from 2.7 to 7.7 per 100,000, a 2.9-fold increase. This has been attributed to several factors, including widespread use of neck ultrasonography and FNA of very small thyroid nodules, improved diagnostic recognition of follicular and other variants of PTC, increased environmental and occupational exposure to ionizing radiation, and increase in iodine-rich (fish, seaweed, iodized salt) diets [15]. Evidence also suggests that benign thyroid diseases, such as chronic lymphocytic (Hashimoto's) thyroiditis, follicular adenoma and Grave's disease are present in an increased number of patients who develop PTC [18]. While PTC generally carries an excellent prognosis some patients develop recurrent and/or metastatic disease with poor outcome.

Approximately 2.5 to 8% of non-medullary thyroid cancers (NMTC, i.e., PTC and FTC) are of familial origin [19]. The majority of kindreds are small and while inheritance patterns appear autosomal dominant, there is a general lack of penetrance of disease. Indeed, variable expression suggests that the responsible inherited genes impart a predisposition or susceptibility to thyroid cancer rather than a cause. In addition, pedigree members of families with familial NMTC are considered to be at increased risk of benign thyroid disease, including follicular adenoma, diffuse and multinodular goiter, and autoimmune thyroiditis. Familial NMTC can be divided into two groups: those with an increased prevalence of NMTC within a familial cancer syndrome characterized by a preponderance of non-thyroidal tumors or those within familial cancer syndromes where the predominant neoplasm is NMTC, although other neoplasms may occur with increased frequency (Familial NMTC Syndrome). The former group includes increased frequency of PTC and FTC in familial adenomatous polyposis (FAP), Carney complex type I, Werner syndrome, multiple endocrine neoplasia (MEN) 2A, and Cowden's syndrome (mostly FTC and rarely PTC). Fewer than 2% of individuals with FAP actually develop PTC but this translates as an increased risk of about 160 times over that of the normal population [20]. Both PTC and FTC are present in about 15% of patients with Carney complex. In Werner syndrome, PTC is the only thyroid neoplasm found in Caucasians whereas FTC and all variants of anaplastic thyroid carcinomas are found in Japanese patients. Microscopic PTC occurs in MEN 2A patients with a frequency that is approximately double that of the normal population. Familial NMTC Syndrome is diagnosed when 2 or more family members have NMTC in the absence of another syndrome. Linkage analysis demonstrates at least four predisposition loci for FNMTC Syndrome in relatively rare extended families, including 1q21 (familial PTC linked to papillary renal neoplasia), 2q21 (FNMTC type 1), 14q31 (familial multinodular goiter syndrome), and 19p13.2 (familial PTC with oxyphilia or Hürthle cell tumors). Definitive evidence of susceptibility genes tied to these loci have yet to be defined [19, 21]. Thyroid histology in these syndromes can be characteristic. For instance, over 90% of patients with FAP who have synchronous PTC, exhibit histologic features of the cribriform-morular variant, a normally very rare subtype of PTC. Such findings should alert the pathologist to the potential need for molecular genetic evaluation of the patient and family members. Generally, FNMTC has a worse prognosis than sporadic forms of the disease, with increased risk of multifocal disease, extrathyroid extension, lymph node metastasis, and recurrence and decreased disease-free survival [18].

Many of the somatic mutations detected in PTC result in constitutive activation of the Ras-Raf-mitogen-activated protein kinase (MAPK)-Erk signalling pathway that is responsible for control of expression of various cellular growth factors involved in proliferation, differentiation, and survival/apoptosis. Indeed, more than 70% of PTC harbor activating point mutations in *BRAF* or Ras genes, or structural chromosomal rearrangements of various tyrosine kinase receptors, including *RET* and *NTRK1* [22,23]. These mutations seem to be mutually exclusive of one another in any given tumor.

BRAF mutations are the most commonly detected abnormality in PTC, seen in roughly 45% of sporadic adult cases but infrequently (0 to 12%) in pediatric and radiation-induced tumors. The V600E mutation occurs in more than 90% of *BRAF*-mutated PTC. Fusion of the N-terminus of *AKAP9* with the C-terminus of *BRAF*, due to a paracentric inversion on 7q, also activates *BRAF* in radiation-associated PTC. *BRAF* mutations are usually found in conventional and tall cell histological variants of PTC, and less frequently in oncocytic/Warthin-like, subcapsular sclerosing, and follicular PTC variants, in poorly differentiated and anaplastic thyroid cancer of papillary origin, and in thyroid lymphomas [24]. Because of the absence of *BRAF* mutations in FTC and extreme rarity in benign hyperplastic nodules, identification of a *BRAF* mutation may help in the diagnosis of PTC [25]. Several studies have sought to improve upon cytologic examination of FNA alone by targeting BRAF mutation in indeterminate or suspicious or non-diagnostic specimens [26, 27, 28]. Adoption of such algorithms may substantially reduce the number of patients who require diagnostic thyroid surgery. This will be discussed further later in this chapter.

Generally, PTC with *BRAF* mutation also portends a worse clinical prognosis than PTC lacking *BRAF* mutation. $BRAF^{V600E}$-positive tumors tend to be associated with aggressive clinicopathologic features, including capsular invasion, extrathyroidal extension, multicentricity, refractoriness/recurrence, and lymph node metastases [27, 29, 30]. Moreover, an association between $BRAF^{V600E}$ and disease-specific survival has been demonstrated [31]. *BRAF* mutations are thought to bestow a degree of radioiodine resistance to these tumors possibly due to reduced expression of the sodium iodide symporter at the basal membrane of thyrocytes. Therefore, identification of a $BRAF^{V600E}$ in cytological samples pre-operatively or in resected tumor post-operatively can aid in patient management [32]. Patients with such high-risk tumors may benefit from more intensive management (optimization of surgical procedures or use of adjuvant therapies) and closer and more frequent follow-up [29]. In a preliminary report, $BRAF^{V600E}$ was detected in 8 of 38 (21%) peripheral blood samples from patients with persistent/recurrent PTC, demonstrating the potential to use the marker to monitor for residual or metastatic disease [33].

Small molecule inhibitors to the mutant form of *BRAF* have been effective in the treatment of melanoma and colorectal cancer. While results of preclinical studies examining the effect of mutant *BRAF* inhibitors on thyroid cancer cell lines were encouraging, the anticancer effects documented in subsequent clinical trials with advanced thyroid cancers were less promising. A $BRAF^{V600E}$ inhibitor, selumetinib, is in phase II trials against radioiodine therapy refractory PTC [34]. Clinical investigations of multi-kinase inhibitors and/or combination with other regimens are currently underway in the treatment of advanced thyroid cancers. Another frequent (20-30%) somatic mutation, found almost exclusively in PTC involves chromosomal rearrangements of *RET* at 10q11.2, whereby *RET* falls under the influence of the promoter of one of at least 15 other separate genes that are constitutively expressed in thyroid follicular cells. *RET* is not normally expressed in thyroid tissues, while the partner genes are ubiquitously expressed.

These rearrangements (inversions and translocations) result in juxtaposition of in the C-terminal region of *RET*, containing the tyrosine kinase domain, to the N-terminal portion of the other protein and aberrant ligand-independent activation of MAPK signalling. The rearrangements are named *RET*/PTC1, RET/PTC2, *RET*/PTC3, etc., depending on the genes involved. A summary of these rearrangements is presented in Table 1. *RET*/PTC1 and *RET*/PTC3 result from paracentric inversions on 10q [22] and are the most common types, accounting for >90% of all *RET* rearrangements [35, 36]. *RET*/PTC1 comprises 60-70% of *RET*/PTC rearrangements while *RET*/PTC3 accounts for 20-30% of RET/PTC-positive cases. *RET*/PTC1-associated tumors, involving *RET* fusion with *CCDC6*, are usually classic-type PTC and microcarcinomas and tend to have a more benign clinical course, whereas those associated with *RET*/PTC3, involving *RET* fusion with *NCOA4*, are more commonly a solid-type PTC and are associated with a more aggressive clinical behavior [36, 37]. *RET*/PTC is more common in PTC in children (~60%) and young adults, and in PTC associated with radiation exposure [38].

The frequency of *RET*/PTC rearrangements in PTC varies significantly worldwide, with the greatest incidence reported in radiation contaminated and iodine-deficient regions. *RET*/PTC-negative cases are more likely to spread through the bloodstream to distant metastatic sites [38]. Assessment of *RET*/PTC rearrangements also shows promise in refining diagnosis of suboptimum cytologic samples [28]. *RET*/PTC rearrangements are usually absent from benign thyroid lesions. However, they can have a heterogeneous distribution within a tumor and may be difficult to identify with molecular techniques if only present in a small proportion or isolated segment of tumor [39]. Reports of the occurrence of *RET*/PTC in Hashimoto's thyroiditis and thyroid follicular adenomas and hyperplastic nodules in several studies have not been confirmed by others and remain controversial [40].

Fusion oncoproteins resulting from 1q paracentric inversions involving the neurotrophic tyrosine kinase I gene (NTRK1) and TPR gene or TPM3 gene or a t(1:3)(q21;q11) translocation involving NTRK1 and TFG genes are found exclusively in a subset of PTC [41]. Collectively, chimeric genes resulting from NTRK1 rearrangements are referred to as TRK. As in RET/PTC gene rearrangements, NTRK1 is not normally expressed in thyroid tissues, while the partner genes are ubiquitously expressed.

Thus, when rearranged, the intracellular tyrosine kinase domain of NTRK1 becomes aberrantly expressed in the fusion oncoprotein, activating the MAPK pathway and contributing to the malignant PTC phenotype [42]. Occurring in 5 to 10% of PTC, these rearrangements are not associated with any particular histologic features. However, TRK may be associated with a more aggressive clinical behavior [43]. Prevalence of TRK also varies considerably between locations and populations.

Point mutations in *NRAS, HRAS,* and *KRAS* genes are seen in approximately 10% of PTC, particularly follicular variant [44]. Ras mutated-PTCs tend to be encapsulated and demonstrate less prominent nuclear features as compared to PTCs lacking Ras mutations. By contrast, follicular variant PTCs with *BRAF* mutations tend to be non-encapsulated and infiltrative [45]. There are conflicting reports of higher [46] and lower [41] rates of lymph node metastasis in Ras-mutated tumors versus PTCs lacking Ras mutations. Much of this variability may be due to differing methods of detection and/or tumor heterogeneity.

Studies using gene expression profiling have largely substantiated the current histologic categorization of PTCs, demonstrating significantly different profiles between classic, follicular and other variants [47]. Several genes have been observed to be up-regulated in PTC, specifically *MET, LGALS3* (galectin-3) and *KRT19* (cytokeratin 19) [48, 49]. The application of immunohistochemical (IHC) methods targeting the protein products of these and other markers will likely define a clinical utility for some in the differential diagnoses of PTC variants.

Several specific microRNA (miRNA) signatures have also been consistently demonstrated in PTCs, including up-regulation of miR-221, miR-222, miR-224, miR-155, miR-187, miR-181b, and miR-146b. By contrast, FTC generally demonstrates up-regulation of miR-221, miR-222, miR-155, miR-187, miR-181b, and miR-224 [50]. Specific miRNA profiles may play a role in the genesis of thyroid carcinomas in general and may prove of significant diagnostic value in the future [51].

Table 1. Rearrangements of Ret and Ntrk protooncogenes in papillary thyroid cancers

Rearrangement	Type of Rearrangement	Partner Gene; Name *
RET-PTC1	inv(10)(q11.2;q21.2)	*CCDC6*; coiled-coil domain containing 6
RET-PTC2	t(10;17)(q11.2;q23)	*PRKAR1A*; protein kinase, cAMP-dependent, regulatory type 1 alpha
RET-PTC3	inv(10)(q11.2;q11) (exon 12 of *RET*)	*NCOA4* ; nuclear receptor coactivator 4
RET-PTC4	inv(10)(q11.2;q11) (exon 11 of *RET*)	*NCOA4*; nuclear receptor coactivator 4
RET-PTC5	t(10;14)(q11.2;q32)	*GOLGA5*; golgin A5
RET-PTC6	t(7;10)(q32-34;q11.2)	*TRIM24*; tripartite motif containing 24
RET-PTC7	t(1;10)(p13.1;q11.2)	*TRIM33*; tripartite motif containing 33
RET-PTC8	t(10;14)(q11.2;q22.1)	*KTN1*; kinectin
RET-PTC9	t(10;18)(q11.2;q21-q22)	*RFG9*
RET-ERC1	t(10;12)(q11.2;p13.3)	*ERC1*; ELKS/RAB6-interacting/CAST family member 1
RET-HOOK3	t(8;10)(p11.21;q11.2)	*HOOK3*; hook homolog 3
RET-TRIM27	t(6;10)(p22;q11.2)	*TRIM27*; tripartite motif containing 27
RET-PCM1	t(8;10)(p21.3-p22;q11.2)	*PCM1*; pericentriolar material 1
NTRK1-T1	inv(1)(q22;q25) (breaks in introns of both genes differ for T1, T2, and T4)	*TPR*; translocated promoter region
NTRK1-T2	inv(1)(q22;q25) (breaks in introns of both genes differ for T1, T2, and T4)	*TPR*; translocated promoter region
NTRK1-T3	t(1;3)(q21-q22;q12.2)	*TFG*; TRK-fused gene
NTRK1-T4	inv(1)(q22;q25) (breaks in introns of both genes differ for T1, T2, and T4)	*TPR*; translocated promoter region
NTRK1-TPM3	inv(1)(q22;q21.2)	*TPM3* (1q21.2); tropomyosin 3

* Gene symbols as per HUGO Gene Nomenclature Committee.

Follicular Thyroid Carcinoma

Follicular thyroid carcinoma is associated with several potential etiologic factors, including iodine deficiency, exposure to ionizing radiation, pre-existing benign thyroid disease (solitary nodule/adenoma and goiter) and several familial syndromes, including Cowden disease, Werner syndrome, and Carney complex I [52, 19]. Thyroid histology in familial PTC syndromes can be characteristic. For instance, FTC in Cowden disease often shows multicentric, well-circumscribed, non-encapsulating, solid, cellular adenomatous nodules, sharing features with follicular adenomas [53]. Such findings should alert the pathologist to the potential need for molecular genetic evaluation of the patient and family members.

A number of somatic alterations have been shown to be involved in the development of follicular cell-derived cancers. Similar to PTC, many of these occur in components of important cell signalling pathways, in particular MAPK signalling. The most common somatic mutations seen in FTC (40-50% of cases) occur within *NRAS*, *HRAS* and *KRAS*; *NRAS* mutations are the most frequent, followed by *HRAS* and *KRAS*. Commonly, amino acid substitutions occur within codons 12, 13, or 61 of the Ras genes. Codon 61 is most frequently affected in NRAS and HRAS and codons 12 and 13 in KRAS. Mutant Ras proteins constitutively activate the Raf-MEK-MAPK and phosphatidylinositol-3-kinase (PI3K)/AKT cell signalling pathways, resulting in dysregulation of specific genes that promote thyroid proliferation and differentiation. Ras mutations are also seen in a significant proportion (20 to 40%) of follicular adenomas [54, 55] but it remains unclear whether these lesions represent preinvasive FTC. Also, Ras mutations are found in about 35% of PDTC and 50% of ATC, where their presence seems to correlate with more aggressive tumor behavior and poor prognosis.

The second most common mutation found in FTC (30 to 40% of cases) involves in-frame fusion of the promoter and DNA binding domains of the thyroid transcription factor *PAX8* with the nuclear receptor domains of the peroxisome proliferator-activated receptor gamma (*PPARγ1*) gene following a t(2;3)(q13;p25) rearrangement. Normal follicular cells express high levels of *PAX8* transcription factor, which is essential for regulating expression of thyroglobulin, thyroperoxidase and the sodium/iodide symporter. PPARγ1 is also a transcription factor that is expressed in normal follicular cells and inhibits cell growth and promotes cell differentiation. The PAX8/PPARγ1-fusion protein results in overexpression of *PPARγ1*, although the exact oncogenic mechanism of action remains unclear [56]. Tumorigenesis also likely involves deregulation of normal PAX8 pathways in thyroid cells via novel fusion protein activities. Immunohistochemical (IHC) staining for PPARγ or t(2;3) detection by fluorescence *in situ* hybridization (FISH) may be useful tools in the diagnosis of malignancy in thyroid follicular lesions. Generally, *PAX8/ PPARγ1* rearrangement and Ras mutations are mutually exclusive, suggesting that tumors harboring these mutations follow different paths of oncogenesis. Tumors with the *PAX8/ PPARγ1* rearrangement tend to have a more solid growth pattern and a higher rate of vascular invasion than tumors without the rearrangement [57], although they also usually carry a more favorable prognosis. Histologically, they demonstrate a morphologic phenotype of microfollicular, solid/trabecular growth, thick fibrous capsule and immunopositivity for galectin-3 and/or HBME-1 [58]. The latter markers have been reported to be occasionally useful in differentiating benign and malignant thyroid tumors. *PAX8/ PPARγ1* rearrangements are also found in 2-10% of follicular adenomas and in follicular variant of PTC but only rarely in conventional PTC [59, 60].

Mutations have also been described in elements of the PI3K signalling pathway within FTCs. This pathway influences gene expression related to cell survival, proliferation, and migration and may be more important in tumor progression than tumorigenesis [61]. The *PIK3CA* gene is mutated in 6 to 13% of FTCs, and gene copy numbers are increased in up to 25% of such tumors [62, 63].

Additionally, mutations in Ras and *PTEN* may impact this pathway. *PTEN* mutations, identified in 6 to 12% of FTC; decrease the inhibitory function of PTEN resulting in activation of AKT and its downstream targets [64].

Gene expression profiling has been applied to follicular tumors, particularly with an aim to identify genetic biomarkers indicative of invasive disease, since this is a particularly challenging component of cytological evaluation of these tumors. Increased expression of three significant genes, *PSCK2, PLAB* and *RAP2A*, was identified in one study; however, of these, only RAP2A (a Ras-related protein) was noted to be significantly increased in invasive FTC compared to encapsulated follicular tumors [65]. Overexpression of normal (non-mutated) c-myc and c-fos has also been reported for FTC and other thyroid neoplasms [66, 67].

Hürthle Cell Thyroid Carcinomas

The molecular bases for the majority of Hürthle cell carcinomas are still largely unknown. Frequently they demonstrate Ras and other mutations shared by FTC, which is consistent with their inclusion as a variant of FTC. However, *RET*/PTC and *BRAF* mutations are also found in these tumors, which are hallmarks of classic PTC. As a result, a separate sub-category of Hürthle cell neoplasms has been proposed, namely the papillary variant. Such papillary variant Hürthle cell tumors have been reported to have a higher incidence of regional metastatic disease [68].

Mutations of nuclear-encoded mitochondrial genes and mitochondrial DNA have also been reported at high frequencies in these tumors [69, 70]. Mutations in *GRIM19* gene, which maps to 19p13.2 and plays a role in assembly of respiratory chain complex I within mitochondria and apoptosis, have been identified with high frequency in some Hürthle cell tumor series but not in others [71]. Such mutations of mitochondrial associated genes may be reflected in the increased number of mitochondria and mitochondrial structural abnormalities that are commonly associated with Hürthle cell neoplasms. Allelic losses at 19p13.2 and 2q21, that are also associated with familial NMTC, are prevalent in Hürthle cell tumors [72]. Gene expression profiling of Hürthle cell thyroid carcinomas and adenomas was used to identify several candidate diagnostic markers that provided sensitivity between 94 and 97% and specificity of 97% for detection of carcinoma [50B]. Overexpression of p53, p27, cyclin D3, N-myc oncogene, tumor growth factor (TGF)-alpha, TGF-beta, insulin-like growth factor (IGF)-1, and somatostatin receptor have also been demonstrated in isolated studies of Hürthle cell carcinomas.

Poorly-Differentiated and Anaplastic Thyroid Carcinomas

Poorly-differentiated (insular) thyroid carcinoma (PDTC) is an uncommon entity, best characterized as a tumor of follicular cells with partial loss of follicular characteristics. Heuristically, these tumors are thought to arise along one of two potential pathways; *de novo* from thyroid follicular epithelium or indirectly by dedifferentiation either from well-differentiated PTC or well-differentiated FTC [74]. These two mechanisms should not be considered mutually exclusive. Evidence for tumor progression through dedifferentiation includes some cases of differentiated NMTC that recurs as PDTC or even anaplastic (undifferentiated) carcinomas (ATC). Also, some differentiated thyroid tumors, particularly of the papillary type, can show evidence of PDTC or ATC and share identical mutations in the various components.

Molecular alterations observed in these tumors include those observed in well-differentiated follicular cell-derived tumors (e.g., *BRAF* and Ras) that probably represent initial molecular events and those viewed as being more specific to poorly-differentiated carcinomas (e.g., *TP53* and beta-catenin (*CTNNB1*)) that probably represent subsequent changes associated with tumor progression. *TP53* mutations are present in about one third of PDTC, and are even more frequent in anaplastic (undifferentiated) carcinomas (ATC), suggesting a role in tumor progression. Demonstration of p53 by IHC frequently correlates with the presence of *TP53* mutation, which is seen in 40-50% of PDTC [75].

Anaplastic carcinoma is a highly aggressive malignancy of the thyroid that has lost most evidence of follicular cell origin. It accounts for less than 2% of thyroid malignancies, although rates vary geographically, and characteristically it occurs in older adults. It is more frequent in individuals with a history of thyroid disease, either benign or malignant, and those with a history of iodine deficiency or radiation exposure [76]. The molecular alterations observed in ATC are similar to those in PDTC, but occur at increased frequency; *TP53* mutations are seen in 50-80% of cases [77] where it leads to dysregulation of apoptosis and cell division, and mutations in the β-catenin gene (*CTNNB1*) seen in up to 65% of cases [78, 79]. The β-catenin protein plays a role in cell adhesion and Wnt signalling. *PTEN* mutations are observed in a minority of cases but *PIK3CA* kinase domain mutations are found in about 15% of ATC and *PIK3CA* copy number gains in up to about 40% of ATC. In contrast with well-differentiated NMTC where *PIK3CA* and *PTEN* mutations rarely coexist with other mutations, *PIK3CA* and *PTEN* mutations are frequently present concurrently with *BRAF* or Ras mutations in ATC.

In one study, $BRAF^{V600E}$ was present in both differentiated and anaplastic components of up to 25% of ATCs whereas *PIK3CA* mutations were primarily localized in anaplastic components only [80]. These findings suggest that *BRAF* mutations play a role in tumorigenesis of at least a subset of ATCs, while *PIK3CA* alterations occur later and are the most relevant events associated with tumor progression. Mutations involving Ras genes have been reported in 6 to 50% of ATC [81, 82].

Several studies have evaluated tumor expression profiles using immunophenotyping of differentiated thyroid cancer (DTC) and ATC as a way to understand the molecular changes that potentially occur during the dedifferentiation process. In one study, 25 of 54 molecular markers tested were significantly differentially expressed between ATC and DTC, and a panel of 5 of these markers readily separated DTC from ATC with a high degree of accuracy [83]. Adoption of such immunophenotyping panels will likely afford beneficial diagnostic and prognostic tools for the management of these and other thyroid lesions.

Medullary Thyroid Carcinoma

The majority of MTC cases are sporadic, but 20-30% are hereditary and demonstrate an autosomal dominant pattern of inheritance. Hereditary cases are classified into three categories: multiple endocrine neoplasia type 2A (MEN 2A), associated with increased risk of pheochromocytoma and parathyroid hyperplasia and/or adenoma; MEN 2B associated with increased risk of pheochromocytoma, mucosal neuromas, gastrointestinal ganglioneuromatosis along with marfanoid body habitus; and familial medullary thyroid carcinoma (FMTC), which is generally seen as a milder subtype of MEN2A. FMTC is often defined as the presence of at least 4 members of a family presenting with MTC without any other signs or symptoms of pheochromocytoma or hyperparathyroidism in the proband or other family members. Germline, gain-of-function point mutations of *RET* that cause activation of MAPK and other signalling pathways governing cell proliferation, survival, and differentiation are found in more than 95% of cases of MEN 2 and 88% of cases of FMTC [84, 85 86]. *RET* is normally expressed on parfollicular C-cells, adrenal medulla, sympathetic ganglia and some other sites [87].

Multiple point mutations have been described, which have been generally ascribed to one of three categories that correlate with age-of-onset and aggressiveness of disease. The majority of MEN 2A and FMTC cases are associated with mutations in the extracellular domains of *RET* and facilitate constitutive dimerization and activation of the intracellular kinase domain. MEN 2B-related *RET* mutations have only been observed in the intracellular domain, which alter the tyrosine kinase conformation within the cell [88]. Since penetrance of these mutations for thyroid cancer is nearly 100%, prophylactic thyroidectomy is the standard intervention for patients who carry a *RET* mutation; timing for this surgery often depends on individual risk assignment. DNA sequencing of select exons or other methods targeting specific mutations of *RET* have been used to detect family members affected by or vulnerable to hereditary MTC and has largely replaced calcitonin monitoring.

Rarely, thyroid tumors with mixed medullary-papillary components or medullary-follicular components have been described. Although recognized as a distinct WHO category [89], studies of this tumor type are usually restricted to individual reports. Specific molecular genetic alterations have not been widely ascribed to tumors in these categories.

Thyroid Lymphomas

Primary thyroid lymphomas are rare, constituting about 5% of all thyroid neoplasms. Practically all these tumors are of the non-Hodgkin type (NHL) with B-cell origin. Although tumors can be aggressive (especially large cell lymphoma) or indolent (low-grade MALT lymphoma), most are highly curable, if diagnosed early and treated correctly. These tumors are frequently found associated with the autoimmune disease Hashimoto thyroiditis, and hypothyroidism [90]. NHL can usually be distinguished from thyroid carcinomas on the basis of immunophenotyping.

Table 2. Major molecular genetic changes associated with thyroid neoplasms

Gene(s)	Associated Tumors	Frequency (%)	Pathway / Point of Action	Benign Lesions
Ras	Follicular Papillary Poorly differentiated Anaplastic	45 10 35 50	MAP Kinase	Adenoma (30%) Nodular goiter (5%)
PAX8/ PPARγ1	Follicular Papillary (FV)	30-40 5	PPARγ1	Adenoma (7%)
GRIM19	Hürthle cell		Apoptosis	
BRAF	Papillary (classic) Poorly differentiated Anaplastic	45 20 20	MAPK, ERK	Adenoma (rare)
RET/PTC	Papillary	20	RTK receptor	
PIK3CA	Follicular Anaplastic	<10 20	PI3K/AKT	
PTEN	Follicular Anaplastic	<10 >10	PI3K/AKT	
TRK	Papillary	<5	NTRK receptor via MAPK	
CTNNB1	Poorly differentiated Anaplastic	20 60		
TP53	Poorly differentiated Anaplastic	20 70	Cell division G1→S	
APC	Papillary	<5		

A significant number of mutations associated with thyroid carcinomas may also be present in primary thyroid lymphomas [91]. Specifically, *BRAF* and *NRAS* mutations have been reported in about 25% and less than 10% of diffuse large B-cell lymphomas, respectively. These findings certainly complicate the differential interpretation based on molecular analyses alone from thyroid FNA samples, but in the context of the morphologic abnormalities usually would not present a problem. See Tables 2 and 3 for a summary of molecular genetic changes associated with various thyroid carcinomas.

**Table 3. Correlation of differentiated thyroid tumor histology
and molecular genetic changes**

Tumor Type	Mutation/ Rearrangement (% Cases)	Morphologic Correlates
Papillary	*BRAF* (45) *RET*/PTC (20) *APC* (<2) Ras (10) *NTRK1* (<5)	Classic type; Tall cell variants PTC1-Classic; PTC3-Solid/micro Cribriform-morular variant Mostly follicular variant
Follicular	Ras (40) *PAX8/ PPARγ1* (30) PIK3CA (<10) *PTEN* (<10) *GRIM19* (<5)	Conventional Solid/microfollicular; Galectin-3/HBME-1 positive Oncocytic
Medullary	*RET* (95% familial, 50% sporadic)	MEN2a/b, FMTC

Detection of Molecular Alterations
in Thyroid Carcinomas

A variety of laboratory methods are available for clinical detection of molecular alterations in thyroid carcinoma specimens. Generally, the testing platforms/techniques employed will be determined by sample type and the type(s) of mutation to be analyzed. PCR-based methods are commonly utilized and provide rapid, reliable and sensitive detection for the spectrum of clinical sample types available, including those of limited quantity, such as FNAs. Qualitative assessment of point mutations in thyroid disease-associated genes can be readily achieved using allele-specific PCR, PCR-RFLP, PCR-melt analysis, PCR-hybridization (including microarrays), Sanger sequencing, pyrosequencing, and other methods [92]. Analytic sensitivity of is an important consideration when validating these assays since involved tumor may represent only a minor component of the available specimen. Moreover, tumors may show considerable heterogeneity in the presence of the mutation being targeted due to clonal evolution processes. Manual gross and microscopic-guided dissection or laser microdissection of tissue section can be used to enrich for tumor cells. Nested- and COLD-PCR methods may also be used to improve analytical sensitivity when the amount of targeted sequences is anticipated to be low in patient specimens. Real-time PCR methods are often used in qualitative assessment of thyroid lesions and generally have the attractive added feature of high analytical sensitivity. By contrast, clinical applications of quantitative real-time PCR for the detection of molecular markers of thyroid cancer are extremely limited; however, such techniques may realize greater utility in the near future for diagnosis/prognosis of thyroid cancer and for monitoring of patients following treatment [93, 94]. In *RET* and other genes, point mutations, deletions and/or insertions associated with thyroid disease processes, can occur at multiple locations; loci can be screened by using multiple singleplexed PCRs combined with some type of conformational analyses of the PCR amplicons (e.g., denaturing HPLC, single-stranded conformational polymorphism, high resolution melt analysis) followed by reflex sequencing of positive samples. Alternatively, more conventional targeted sequencing of specific loci or multiplexed-PCR approaches can be undertaken.

Detection of chromosomal rearrangements in thyroid carcinomas, such as *RET*/PTC or *PAX8/ PPARγ1*, usually demand the use of reverse-transcriptase PCR (RT-PCR) or fluorescence *in-situ* hybridization (FISH) approaches to analysis. Since the breakpoints in such chromosomal rearrangements may occur over considerable genetic distances, the analyte of choice for PCR-based analyses is RNA, which lacks the extensive intronic sequences present in genomic DNA. This often necessitates duteous attention to the collection and processing of specimens (generally, fresh or snap-frozen FNAs and surgical biopsies) and coordination with surgical and pathology staff to assure optimal preservation of RNA for the downstream RT-PCR analysis. Otherwise, thyroid tissues are processed by routine formalin-fixation and paraffin embedding (FFPE), which may compromise the possibility of some RT-PCR analyses. By contrast, interphase FISH can be effectively used to detect many chromosomal rearrangements in FFPE thyroid tissues or other nodules.

Given the paucity of FDA-approved *in vitro* diagnostic tests for thyroid cancer and the potential impact that a positive test result has in the clinical management of patients, all laboratory-developed tests must be subject to rigorous validation to assure highly specific, sensitive and reproducible results. While there is often a desire to be able to detect low numbers of cells that carry the disease causing mutation, this must be tempered with the realization that increased false-positivity will accompany ultrasensitive detection methods. For instance, in one study using dual-priming oligonucleotide (DPO)-based multiplex PCR analysis, which was estimated to detect $BRAF^{V600E}$ in 2% of cells within a background of wild-type cells, false-positive results were revealed in five of 226 (2%) FNAs tested [95]. Reproducibility testing is essential in establishing clinically relevant cut-off values for all these tests. For interphase FISH, sectioning of FFPE tissues often results in nuclei with less than the full complement of probe signals. Moreover, signal patterns also may vary with section thickness. Therefore, appropriate cut-off values need to be carefully established during the validation of these tissue-based assays.

Several commercial products have been developed to aid in the clinical diagnosis of thyroid cancers. One approach employs micro-array evaluation of the expression profiles of 142 genes involved in various biologic pathways, including some markers of thyroid lesions detailed in the preceding sections as well as some not previously implicated in cancer [96]. This initial analysis is followed by a proprietary algorithm whereby the expression profile observed for a given patient is compared to a molecular classifier database. Validation of the original dataset used to establish the molecular classifier involved comparison of expression profiles of cytologic and surgical biopsies to histopathologic diagnoses rendered by a panel of expert pathologists. The molecular classifier claims a sensitivity of 95% and specificity of 63% for indeterminate cytology samples and 97% and 64%, respectively, for all samples. Proteomic detection of mutation status through commonly available clinical platforms such as immunohistochemistry is also a possibility going forward. To this end, the recent report describing successful detection of $BRAF^{V600E}$ –mutated protein appears promising [97]. Similarly, in other organ systems, p53 immunohistochemistry findings have been shown to correspond to $TP53$ mutation status [98].

Clinical Application of Molecular Testing

Application of molecular testing introduces potentially costly and complex additional processes to what has been a relatively simple cascade of clinical and pathologic evaluations, albeit a somewhat flawed cascade considering the high proportion of potentially avoidable surgical outcomes. The financial practicality and effectiveness of integrating molecular testing into the algorithm is, in part, dependent on the cost of this added laboratory testing weighed against the savings accrued due to surgical and other over-treatment-related costs versus any added expenditures from adverse outcomes due to under-treatment. This cost-benefit evaluation will differ according to the numbers of patients in a given cytologic category and the relative risk of malignancy in that category. Since multiple genetic markers are often evaluated any one case, this cost is not trivial.

Since the risk of malignancy in cytologically-negative samples is less than 3%, there is little impetus to perform pre-operative molecular testing on these patients at this time. Similarly, in samples categorized as positive for malignancy, further molecular testing with diagnostic intent is superfluous, though it may be considered for other reasons mentioned below, as malignancy is confirmed in this setting in 97-98% of cases. Cytologic accuracy in interpretation of thyroid aspirates is observer dependent, particularly in the borderline categories where the kappa statistic for interobserver agreement are as low as 0.11, a factor which should remain in consideration when evaluating the specificity of molecular analyses or a reflex algorithm [99]. However, in terms of critical management decision cut-offs, the cytology kappa statistics are good (0.72), a result in part attributable to efforts in standardization and education such as the Bethesda System [100].

Positive results for *BRAF* mutation in atypical or indeterminate cytology samples can be virtually diagnostic of PTC [101, 102]. Likewise, clonal rearrangement of *RET*/PTC is also reasonably specific for PTC. Ras mutations are not specific for PTC or FTC, nor indeed for carcinoma, as they are also found in a number of benign conditions. But the presence of this alteration in association with other clinical or cytological features may be useful in directing further therapy. For example, Ras mutations found in a cytologically classified "follicular lesion" could represent a follicular variant of PTC, or a follicular adenoma. But since this mutation may predispose a patient to progression of adenoma to follicular carcinoma, surgical removal of such adenomas may be appropriate. In addition, the presence of *BRAF* mutation in thyroid tumors has prognostic and therapeutic implications; *BRAF* mutation is associated with increased aggressiveness and lack of response of recurrences to radioiodine due to impaired iodine trapping mechanisms as discussed earlier in this chapter [103]. Moreover, novel targeted therapies to *BRAF* have been used with limited success in advanced thyroid carcinomas [104]. In some studies, the positive predictive value of *BRAF, RET*/PTC and *PAX8/ PPARγ1* has been found to be 100% for PTC or FTC. Ras mutations also have a high positive predictive value at 87.5%, and carry the additional value of being positive in cytologic situations that are more challenging, i.e. follicular variants of PTC and FTC [28]. Thus a panel of molecular tests that includes *BRAF, RET*/PTC, Ras and *PAX8/ PPARγ1* has been advocated for evaluation of cytologic samples with indefinite findings for malignancy as a means of more reliably categorizing these patients. The data (see Table 4) tend to support this application especially for those specimens categorized as "follicular lesion of uncertain significance" (FLUS) [105]. A more recent, larger study by the same group using nearly a thousand cytologic samples from over 500 patients found that the detection of any mutation in their panel conferred a risk of histologic malignancy ranging from 88-95% for cytologic samples in the indeterminate categories [106]. Still significant numbers of malignancies remain within the mutation-negative, "follicular lesion" and "suspicious for malignancy" groups. In fact, in the same study, the risk of malignancy in these same categories ranged from 6-28%. Only in the samples categorized as "atypia of unknown significance/follicular lesion of undetermined significance" did the negative predictive value of mutation analysis exceed a 90% threshold that might offer comfort in "watchful waiting" as follow-up. Another study using a similar panel, but with the addition of assays for *TRK* mutation, found a combined negative predictive value (NPV) of cytology and molecular analysis of up to 96%, although their study did not uncover any *TRK* or *PPARγ1* mutation-positive cases [107]. This high NPV is based on including mutation-positive cases which ultimately proved to be adenoma as "true" positives. Their study selected patients who were undergoing surgery regardless of the outcome however, so this selection biased population may not truly represent all patients presenting with thyroid nodules for cytologic evaluation.

Further methodologic means have been sought to improve the NPV using next generation sequencing (NGS) and gene expression profiling for an expanded array of potentially significant markers beyond the known mutations we have described. The commercially available Affirma panel uses the expression profile of 142 genes and a proprietary algorithm to prospectively assign nodules (based on testing of samples obtained by FNA) into a benign or suspicious category [108]. The performance characteristics of this test have been reported as having a NPV of 95%, 94% and 85% for cytologic samples reported as FLUS/AUS, FN/SFN, and Suspicious for malignancy (SMC) respectively [108A]. Salmon's group in Bruxelles utilized a validated "hotspot" NGS panel to evaluate 34 cytologic samples with increased risk of malignancy. In their hands, this method had a NPV of 92%, with a PPV of 63%, still lower than ideal to inspire willing "watchful waiting" for patients with a negative test. [108B] Others who have used NGS in evaluation of potential thyroid neoplasm have also found it an effective method for detecting tumor-related mutations, including some additional somatic mutations involving the TSHR gene and GNAS, but also report a NPV that still falls below 95% [108C, 106]

In practical terms this means that the clinical management of molecular marker-negative patients with borderline FNA results is not significantly impacted, although the type of surgery offered might differ (lobectomy vs. total thyroidectomy). However, Nikiforov and colleagues also found evidence that management of mutation analysis-positive patients can be favorably impacted by pre-surgical knowledge of the mutation type that is present [106]. This could potentially reduce the number of patients in the molecular-positive group who would require two procedures for proper management of their cancer. Whether this impact will outweigh the costs of testing all FNA samples requires further study.

Table 4. Cytologic classification and associated risk of malignancy

Cytologic Category	% With Malignancy (Cytology only)	% With Malignancy If Positive Molecular Marker	Notes
Unsatisfactory	0		
Negative	2-10	100	0.9% if negative [53]
FLUS	5-10	100	No cancers in mutation negative group (n=21)
Follicular lesion	20-30	100	21% cancers in mutation negative group (n=23)
Suspicious for malignancy	50-75	100	50% (n=7)
Positive for malignancy	98	100	

Adapted from data from Nikiforov et al [105].

These data illustrate (again) the importance of sensitivity along with specificity in any testing algorithm and ensuring that study sample selection is comparable to clinical usage patterns. Cytology alone is quite sensitive in detecting follicular-cell derived neoplasms. It is quite specific in classifying those cases not needing further evaluation, i.e., a high negative predictive value. A molecular panel as noted above has a very high specificity for malignant lesions, but does yet not have a particularly good negative predictive value, when applied to the group of cytologically indeterminate cases.

Consideration is being given also to adding miRNA evaluation to the panel of mutation markers described above, in the hopes of further improving the negative predictive value to a clinically usable level but solid data to form action is yet to appear. As mentioned previously, an alternative approach, also directed at indeterminate cytologic samples, based on evaluation of mRNA as a marker of gene expression, is currently marketed by a for-profit venture, and validated by a number of participating academic and private institutions in the USA [108, 109]. Early studies using this proprietary assay and algorithm have shown a high negative predictive value for the results, and theoretical claims of cost-effectiveness based on routine use with indeterminate cytology findings [110]. Also, serum biomarker approaches to the evaluation of thyroid carcinoma (discussed below) show promise [111].

Use of traditional immunohistochemical assays as a means of further clarifying the differential diagnosis is sometimes possible with sufficient cytologic material. Because most clinical laboratories are familiar with immunocytochemistry and immunohistochemistry, protein-based assays have a great potential for clinical use. Galectin-3 (Gal-3), Hector Battifora mesothelial cell-1 monoclonal antibody (HBME-1), cytokeratin 19 (CK19), C-X-C ligand receptor 4 (CXCR4), and insulin-like growth factor mRNA binding protein 3 (IMP3), Met, and hepatocyte growth factor have been investigated as potential markers for IHC evaluation of indeterminate thyroid cytologies [112, 113, 114, 115]. Combination profiles of these with newer mutation-specific antibodies may eventually play a role in evaluation, but cannot currently be recommended.

Application of non-mutation specific testing to indeterminate cytologic samples may also play a future role. Several RNA-based markers have been proposed for inclusion in such panels to differentiate high-risk thyroid lesions. Ubiquitin-conjugating enzyme E2C (UBE2C or UbcH10) is associated with loss of cell-cycle cyclins and has been found to be associated with several tumors. In a study of FNA samples classified as follicular lesion or suspicious for malignancy, the marker was found (both by IHC and quantitative RT-PCR) to have excellent sensitivity for a potentially significant thyroid lesion [116]. High-mobility group AT-hook 2 (HGMA2), a transcription factor, has also been found expressed in adult tumors, including thyroid cancer. Using RT-PCR retrospectively on a group of patients with cytologically suspicious nodules, Lappinga et al. found good sensitivity and high specificity for malignancy in a group of cases that included PTC, FC and Hürthle cell carcinomas, although the latter did not express the marker as highly as the other malignancies [117]. Human telomerase reverse transcriptase (hTERT) has also been suggested as a potential diagnostic marker for thyroid cancer, since this protein is not expressed in most somatic cells, but reappears in many cancers. However, its specificity in the thyroid has been questioned as it may appear in cases of thyroiditis as well [118].

The "positive for malignancy" cytologic category will include both differentiated thyroid carcinomas of papillary type and medullary type, together with poorly-differentiated and anaplastic tumor types. Generally, the latter two categories will not benefit significantly from further molecular testing in terms of diagnosis or prognosis. If a medullary carcinoma is recognized cytologically as an index case, further evaluation of blood or tumor from the patient for germline *RET* mutations can be useful if other family members are to be screened. Prospective studies to evaluate the further utility of *PTEN* or *NTRK1* mutations have not been applied to cytologic samples. However, given the relatively low prevalence of these mutations, the expected added value of these assays would appear to be low. If the *BRAF* mutation IHC stain is ultimately found to have the stellar performance noted in the preliminary studies, this might also have a consistent role in this category to help guide the type of surgical procedure selected.

Application of molecular testing to surgical pathology specimens has some added value in the setting of an atypical thyroid follicular lesion with patchy or focal features suggesting PTC, where other methods (IHC and routine HandE) are inconclusive. Demonstration of a mutation such as Ras, *RET*/PTC or *BRAF* might support making the diagnosis of carcinoma and giving further appropriate treatment. Encapsulated lesions like this have consistently been shown to contain the mutation, even though the cytologic alterations are present only focally. Another use of molecular evaluation in surgical pathology might be in directing therapy more individually. Being able to use *BRAF*-mutation status to predict responsiveness to conventional radioiodine treatment or to a specific targeted therapeutic agent could be a valuable adjunct to traditional diagnostic reporting.

Our improved understanding of the molecular pathogenesis and progression of thyroid lesions has allowed studies of novel targeted agents to be carried out on thyroid cancer patients and provided much needed therapeutic options to those with advanced disease. Multiple clinical trials utilizing tyrosine kinase inhibitors (TKIs), such as sorafenib, sunitinib, selumetinib, imatinib, axitinib, and motesanib diphosphate, and vandetanib, have shown varying responses to follicular, papillary, anaplastic, and medullary thyroid carcinomas [115, 119]. Vandetanib has become standard of care for treatement of symptomatic or progressive MTC, based on significantly improved progression-free survival in clinical trials [120]. Individual TKIs often exert their effect on multiple cellular pathways, including tyrosine kinases, tyrosine kinase receptors and their ligands (e.g., vascular endothelial growth factor receptor), thereby potentially providing a basis for the treatment of biologically divergent thyroid tumors. Other novel non-TKI agents have also been used in phase I or II settings for advanced thyroid cancers and the number of options and trials continues to expand [88, 121]. As targeted therapies move from clinical trials phases to mainstream use, knowledge of mutation status will likely be recommended, or required as part of the FDA initiative for companion drug testing, to establish drug-eligibility.

Conclusion

The distinct, and largely mutually exclusive, mutation pathways observed in PTC (mostly *RET*/Ras/*BRAF*/MAPK) versus FTC (mostly due to mutations of Ras or *PAX8/PPARγ1* translocation) provides an opportunity to use various molecular markers in improving diagnostic accuracy. However, the clinical sensitivity and specificity of individual markers are often too low to provide clinical utility as the combined negative predictive values leave significant clinical gaps in management. The evaluation of indeterminate thyroid FNA cytologic samples with a panel of molecular tests shows significant promise in allowing further risk-stratification for presence of malignancy and thus potentially reducing needless surgery. The probability of malignancy for patients with an indeterminate FNA cytology is about 40% [14]. A molecular panel of tests including *BRAF*, *PAX8/PPARγ1*, Ras, and *RET* is able to identify a group of patients with virtually 100% probability of malignancy, thus helping to expedite them towards surgical or other therapies. However, in using such a molecular panel, up to 30% of thyroid cancers will have no mutation detected, a proportion too high to ignore clinically. Hence, what to do with indeterminate cytologic samples that are negative for the panel of molecular tests we have identified remains a challenge. A testing algorithm with a very high negative predictive value for patients with indeterminate cytologic findings is still needed in order to inspire confidence in the path of watchful waiting or inaction.

Preoperative identification of mutation status is likely to partly guide surgical treatment of PTC, as well as additional treatment options for surgically resected thyroid malignancies. In the era of targeted therapy, mutation status will become as important a piece of data as histologic type.

References

[1]   Howlader N, Noone AM, Krapcho M, Neyman N, Aminou R, Altekruse SF, Kosary CL, Ruhl J, Tatalovich Z, Cho H, Mariotto A, Eisner MP, Lewis DR, Chen HS, Feuer EJ, Cronin KA (eds). *SEER Cancer Statistics Review,* 1975-2009 (Vintage 2009 Populations), National Cancer Institute. Bethesda, MD. http://seer.cancer.gov/csr/1975_2009_ pops09/, based on November 2011 SEER data submission, posted to the SEER web site 2012.

[2]   National Cancer Institute, *A Snapshot of Head and Neck and Thyroid Cancers,* http://www.cancer.gov/aboutnci/servingpeople/snapshots/head-neck.pdf [Accessed 22 Mar 2011].

[3]   Kushchayeva Y, Duh QY, Kebebew E, Clark OH. Prognostic indications for Hürthle cell cancer. *World J. Surg.,* Dec 2004, 28(12):1266-70.

[4]   Neff RL, Farrar WB, Kloos RT, Burman KD. Anaplastic thyroid cancer. *Endocrinol. Metab. Clin. North Am.,* Jun 2008, 37(2):525-38, xi.

[5]   Kebebew E; Greenspan FS; Clark OH; Woeber KA; McMillan A et al. Anaplastic thyroid carcinoma. *Cancer,* 2005 Apr 1, 103(7):1330-5.

[6]   Nabriski D, Ness-Abramof R, Brosh TO, et al. Clinical relevance of non-palpable thyroid nodules as assessed by ultrasound-guided fine needle aspiration biopsy. *J. Endocrinol. Invest.,* Jan 2003, 26(1):61-64.

[7]   Van Nostrand D. Radionuclide imaging of thyroid nodules. In: *Thyroid Cancer,* 2006, Part III (pp. 223-228) DOI: 10.1007/978-1-59259-995-0_20.

[8]   Mandel SJ. Diagnostic use of ultrasonography in patients with nodular thyroid disease. *Endocr. Pract.,* May-Jun 2004, 10(3):246-252.

[9]   Miller JM, Hamburger JI, Kini S. Diagnosis of thyroid nodules. Use of fine-needle aspiration and needle biopsy. *JAMA,* 1979, 241:481-484.

[10] Prinz RA, O'Morchoe PJ, Barbato AL, et al. Fine needle aspiration biopsy of thyroid nodules. *Ann. Surg.,* 1983, 198:70-73.

[11] Gharib H, Goellner JR. Fine-needle aspiration biopsy of the thyroid: an appraisal. *Ann. Intern. Med.,* 1993, 118:282-289.

[12] Baloch ZW, Cibas ES, Clark DP, Layfield LJ, Ljung B, Pitman MB, Abati A. The National Cancer Institute thyroid fine needle aspiration state of the science conference: A summation. *Cyto Journal,* 2008, 5:6.

[13] Theoharis CG, Schofield KM, Hammers L, Udelsman R, Chhieng DC. The Bethesda thyroid fine-needle aspiration classification system: year 1 at an academic institution. *Thyroid,* 2009 Nov, 19(11):1215-1223.

[14] Nayar R, Ivanovic M. The indeterminate thyroid fine-needle aspiration: experience from an academic center using terminology similar to that proposed in the 2007 National Cancer Institute Thyroid Fine Needle Aspiration State of the Science Conference. *Cancer Cytopathol.,* 2009 Jun 25, 117(3):195-202.

[15] Danese D, Sciacchitano S, Farsetti A, Andreoli M, Pontecorvi A. diagnostic accuracy of conventional versus sonography-guided fine-needle aspiration biopsy of thyroid nodules. *Thyroid,* 1998, 8(1):15-21.

[16] Cesur M, Corapcioglu D, Bulut S, Gursoy A, Yilmaz AE, Erdogan N, Kamel N. Comparison of palpation-guided fine-needle aspiration biopsy to ultrasound-guided fine-needle aspiration biopsy in the evaluation of thyroid nodules. *Thyroid,* 2006, 16(6):555-561.

[17] Yokozawa T, Fukata S, Kuma K, Matsuzuka F, Kobayashi A, Hirai K, Miyauchi A, Sugawara M. Thyroid cancer detected by ultrasound-guided fine-needle aspiration biopsy. *World J. Surg.,* 1996, 20(7):848-853.

[18] Nikiforov Y, Ohori P. Papillary carcinoma. In: Nikiforov, Biddinger and Thompson, editors. *Diagnostic Pathology and Molecular Genetics of the Thyroid.* Baltimore, MD: Wolters-Kluwer LWW; 2009; 160-162.

[19] Bonora E, Tallini G, Romeo G. Genetic predisposition to familial nonmedullary thyroid cancer: An update of molecular findings and state-of-the-art studies. *Journal of Oncology*, Volume 2010 (2010), Article ID 385206, 7 pages, doi:10.1155/2010/385206.

[20] Plail RO, Bussey HJ, Glazer G, et al. Adenomatous polyposis: an association with carcinoma of the thyroid. *Br. J. Surg.,* 1987,74:377-380.

[21] Tran T, Gianoukakis AG. Familial thyroid neoplasia: impact of technological advances on detection and monitoring. *Curr. Opin. Endocrinol. Diabetes Obes.,* 2010, 17: 425-431.

[22] Frattini M, Farrario C, Bressan P, et al. Alternative mutations of BRAF, RET and NTRK1 are associated with similar but distinct gene expression patterns in papillary thyroid cancer. *Oncogene,* 2004, 23:7436-7440.

[23] Kimura ET, Nikiforova MN, Zhu Z, et al. High prevalence of BRAF mutations in thyroid cancer: genetic evidence for constitutive activation of RET/PTC-RAS-BRAF signalling pathway in papillary thyroid carcinoma. *Cancer Res.,* 2003, 63:1454-1457.

[24] Yip L, Nikiforova MN, Carty SE, et al. Optimizing surgical treatment of papillary thyroid carcinoma associated with BRAF mutation. *Surgery,* 2009, 146:1215-1223.

[25] Melck AL, Yip L, Carty SE. The utility of BRAF testing in the management of papillary thyroid cancer. *The Oncologist*, December 2010, vol. 15 no. 12 1285-1293.

[26] Jo YS, Huang S, Kim YJ, et al. Diagnostic value of pyrosequencing for the BRAF V600E mutation in ultrasound-guided fine-needle aspiration biopsy samples of thyroid incidentalomas. *Clin. Endocrinol.* (Oxf), 2009, 70:139-144.

[27] Xing M, Tufano RP, Tufaro AP, et al. Detection of BRAF mutation on fine needle aspiration biopsy specimens: A new diagnostic tool for papillary thyroid cancer. *J. Clin. Endocrinol. Metab.,* 2004, 89:2867-2872.

[28] Nikiforov YE, Steward DL, Robinson-Smith TM, et al. Molecular testing for mutations in improving the fine-needle aspiration diagnosis of thyroid nodules. *J. Clin. Endocrinol. Metab.*, 2009, 94:2092-2098.

[29] Nikiforova MN, Kumura ET, Gandhi M, et al. BRAF mutations in thyroid tumors are restricted to papillary carcinomas and anaplastic or poorly differentiated carcinomas arising from papillary carcinomas. *J. Clin. Endocrinol. Metab.*, 2003, 88:5399-5404.

[30] Lupi C, Giannini R, Ugolini C, et al. Association of BRAF V600E mutation with poor clinicopathological outcomes in 500 consecutive cases of papillary thyroid carcinoma. *J. Clin. Endocrinol. Metab.*, 2007, 92:4085-4090.

[31] Finkelstein A, Levy GH, Hui P, et al. Papillary thyroid carcinomas with and without BRAF V600E are morphologically distinct. *Histopathol.*, 2012, 60:1052-1059.

[32] Elisei R, Ugolini C, Viola D, et al. BRAF(V600E) mutation and outcome of patients with papillary thyroid carcinoma: A 15-year median follow-up study. *J. Clin. Endocrinol. Metab.*, 2008, 93:3943-3949.

[33] Cradic KW, Milosevic D, Rosenberg AM, Erickson LA, McIver B, Grebe SK. Mutant BRAF(T1799A) can be detected in the blood of papillary thyroid carcinoma patients and correlates with disease status. *J. Clin. Endocrinol. Meta,*. 2009, 94(12):5001.

[34] Antonelli A, Fallahi P, Ulisse S, et al. New targeted therapies for anaplastic thyroid cancer. *Anticancer Agents Med. Chem.*, 2012, 12(1): 87-93.

[35] NIkiforov Y, Ohori P. op cit p. 164.

[36] Nikiforov Y, Rowland JM, Bove KE, et al. Distinct pattern of ret oncogene rearrangements in morphological variants of radiation-induced and sporadic thyroid papillary carcinomas in children. *Cancer Res.,* 1997, 57:1690-1694.

[37] Santoro M, Melillo RM, Fusco A. RET/PTC activation in papillary thyroid carcinoma. *Eur. J. Endocrinol.*, 2006, 155(5):645-653.

[38] Romei C, Elisei R. RET/PTC translocations and clinico-pathological features in human papillary thyroid carcinoma. *Front Endocrinol.*, 2012, 3:54. http://www.ncbi.nlm.nih. gov/pmc/articles/PMC3356050/.

[39] Zhu Z, Ciampi R, Nikiforova MN, et al. Prevalence of RET/PTC rearrangements in thyroid papillary carcinomas: effects of the detection methods and genetic heterogeneity. *J. Clin. Endocrinol. Metab.*, 2006, 91:3603-3610.

[40] Rhoden KJ, Unger K, Salvatore G, et al. RET/papillary thyroid cancer rearrangement in nonneoplastic thyrocytes: follicular cells of Hashimoto's thyroiditis share low-level recombination events with a subset of papillary carcinoma. *J. Clin. Endocrinol. Metab.*, 2006 Jun, 91(6): 2414-23.

[41] Pierotti MA, Bongarzone I, Borello MG, et al. Cytogenetics and molecular genetics of carcinomas arising from thyroid epithelial follicular cells. *Genes Chromosomes Cancer*, 1996, 16:1-14.

[42] Russell JP, Powell DJ, Cunnane M, et al. The TRK-T1 fusion protein induces neoplastic transformation of thyroid epithelium. *Oncogene,* 2000, 19:5729-5735.

[43] I. Bongarzone, P. Vigneri, L. Mariani, P. Collini, S. Pilotti, and M. A. Pierotti, "RET/NTRK1 rearrangements in thyroid gland tumors of the papillary carcinoma family: correlation with clinicopathological features," *Clinical Cancer Research*, 1998, vol. 4, no. 1, pp. 223–228.

[44] Zhu Z, Gandhi M, Nikiforovna MN, et al. Molecular profile and clinical-pathologic features of the follicular variant of papillary thyroid carcinoma. An unusually high prevalence of ras mutations. *Am. J. Clin. Pathol.,* 2003, 120:71-77.

[45] Rivera M, Ricarte-Filho J, Knauf J, et al. Molecular genotyping of papillary thyroid carcinoma follicular variant according to its histological subtypes (encapsulated vs infiltrative) reveals distinct BRAF and RAS mutation patterns. *Modern Pathol.,* 2010, 23:1191-1200.

[46] Hara H, Fulton N, Yashiro T, et al. N-ras mutation: an independent prognostic factor for aggressiveness of papillary thyroid carcinoma. *Surgery,* 1994, 116:1010-1016.

[47] Giordano TJ, Kuick R, Thomas DG, et al. Molecular classification of papillary carcinoma: distinct BRAF, RAS and RET/PTC mutation-specific gene expression profiles discovered by DNA microarray analysis. *Oncogene,* 2005, 24:6646-6656.

[48] Barbara Jarząb, Małgorzata Wiench, Krzysztof Fujarewicz, Krzysztof Simek, Michał Jarząb, Małgorzata Oczko-Wojciechowska, Jan Włoch, Agnieszka Czarniecka, Ewa Chmielik, Dariusz Lange, Agnieszka Pawlaczek, Sylwia Szpak, Elżbieta Gubała, Andrzej Świerniak Gene expression profile of papillary thyroid cancer: sources of variability and diagnostic implications. *Cancer Res.,* February 15, 2005, 65; 1587.

[49] Chevillard S, Ugolin N, Vielh P, et al. Gene expression profiling of differentiated thyroid neoplasms: diagnostic and clinical implications. *Clin. Cancer Res.,* 204 10:6586-6597.

[50] Chen YT, Kitabayashi N, Zhou XT, et al. MicroRNA analysis as a potential diagnostic tool for papillary thyroid carcinoma. *Mod. Pathol.,* 2008, 21:1139-1146.

[51] Nikiforova MN, Tseng GC, Steward D, et al. MicroRNA expression profiling of thyroid tumors: biological significance and diagnostic utility. *J. Clin. Endocrinol. Metab.,* 2008, 93:1600-1608.

[52] Nikiforov YE, Ohori NP. Follicular carcinoma. In: Nikiforov, Biddinger and Thompson, editors. *Diagnostic Pathology and Molecular Genetics of the Thyroid.* Baltimore, MD: Wolters-Kluwer, LWW; 2009; 132-133.

[53] Harach HR, Soubeyran I, Brown A, et al. Thyroid pathologic findings in patients with Cowden disease. *Ann. Diagn. Pathol.,* 1999, 3:331-340.

[54] Kondo, T., S. Ezzat, and S.L. Asa, Pathogenetic mechanisms in thyroid follicular-cell neoplasia. *Nat. Rev. Cancer,* 2006, 6(4):292-306.

[55] Nikiforova, M.N. and Y.E. Nikiforov, Molecular diagnostics and predictors in thyroid cancer. *Thyroid,* 2009, 19(12):1351-61.

[56] Eberhard NL, Grebe SKG, McIver B, et al. The role of the PAX8/PPARγ fusion oncogene in the pathogenesis of follicular thyroid cancer. *Mol. Cell Endocrinol.,* 2010, 32:50-56.

[57] French CA, Alexander EK, Cibas ES, et al. Genetic and biological subgroups of low-stage follicular thyroid cancer. *Am. J. Pathol.,* 2003, 162: 1053-1060.

[58] Nikiforov MN, Lynch RA, Biddinger PW, et al. RAS point mutations and PAX8/PPAR-gamma rearrangement in thyroid tumors: evidence for distinct molecular pathways in thyroid follicular carcinoma. *J. Clin. Endocrinol. Metab.,* 2003, 88:2318-2326.

[59] Marques, A.R., et al., Expression of PAX8-PPAR gamma 1 rearrangements in both follicular thyroid carcinomas and adenomas. *J. Clin. Endocrinol. Metab.,* 2002, 87(8):3947-52.

[60] Castro, P., et al., PAX8-PPARgamma rearrangement is frequently detected in the follicular variant of papillary thyroid carcinoma. *J. Clin. Endocrinol. Metab.,* 2006, 91(1):213-20.

[61] Shinohara M, Chung YJ, Saji M, et al. AKT in thyroid tumorigenesis and progression. *Endocrinology,* 2007, 148:942-947.

[62] Wang Y, Hou P, Yu H, et al. High prevalence and mutual exclusivity of genetic alterations in the phosphatidylinositol-3-kinase/akt pathway in thyroid tumors. *J. Clin. Endocrinol. Metab.,* 2007, 92: 2387 - 3290.

[63] Wu G, Mambo E, Guo Z, et al. Uncommon mutation, but common amplifications of the PIK3CA gene in thyroid tumors. *J. Clin. Endocrinol. Metab.,* 2005, 90:4688-4693.

[64] Halachmi N, Halachmi S, Evron E, et al. Somatic mutations of the PTEN tumor suppressor gene in sporadic follicular thyroid tumors. *Genes Chromosomes Cancer,* 1998, 23:239-243.

[65] Prabakaran I, Grau JR, Lewis R, et al. Rap2A is upregulated in invasive cells dissected from follicular thyroid cancer. *J. Thyroid Res.,* 2011, 979849, doi:10.4061/2011/979840.

[66] Karga H, Lee JK, Vickery AL, Thor A, Gaz RD, Jameson JL et al: Ras oncogene mutations in benign and malignant thyroid neoplasms. *J. Clin. Endocrinol. Metab.,* 1991, Oct;73(4): 832-836.

[67] Terrier P, Sheng ZM, Schlumberger M, Tubiana M, Cailou B, Travagli JP, Fragu P, Parmentier C et al: Structure and expression of c-myc and c-fos proto-oncogenein thyroid carcinomas. *Br. J. Cancer,* 1988 Jan, 57(1) 43-47.

[68] Maxwell EL, Palme CE, Freeman J. Hürthle cell tumors: applying molecular markers to define a new management algorithm. *Arch. Otolaryngol. Head Neck Surg.,* Jan 2006, 132(1):54-8.

[69] Máximo V, Sobrinho-Simões M. Hürthle cell tumours of the thyroid. A review with emphasis on mitochondrial abnormalities with clinical relevance. *Virchows Arch.* Aug 2000, 437(2):107-15.

[70] Fusco A, Viglietto G, Santoro M. Point mutation in GRIM-19: a new genetic lesion in Hürthle cell thyroid carcinomas. *Br. J. Cancer,* 2005 May 23, 92(10):1817–1818.

[71] Maximo V, Botelho T, Capela J, et al. Somatic and germline mutation in GRIM-19, a dual function gene involved in mitochondrial metabolism and cell death, is linked to mitochondrion-rich (Hürthle cell) tumours of the thyroid. *Br. J. Cancer,* 2005, 92:1892-1898.

[72] Fusco A, Viglietto G, Santoro M. Point mutation in GRIM-19: a new genetic lesion in Hürthle cell thyroid carcinomas. *Br. J. Cancer,* 2005 May 23, 92(10):1817–1818.

[73] Cerutti JM, Oler G, Delcelo R, Gerardt R, Michaluart Jr. P, de Souza SJ, Galante PAF, Huang P, Riggins GJ. PVALB, a new Hürthle adenoma diagnostic marker identified through gene expression. *The Journal of Clinical Endocrinology and Metabolism,* January 1, 2011, 96(1):E151-E160.

[74] Rosai J, Carcangiu ML, DeLellis RA. *Tumors of the Thyroid Gland.* Washington, DC: Armed Forces Institute of Pathology; 1992.

[75] Dobashi Y, Sugimura H, Sakamoto A, et al. Stepwise participation of p53 gene mutation during dedifferentiation of human thyroid carcinomas. *Diagn. Mol. Pathol.,* 1994, 3:9-14.

[76] Seethala RR, Nikiforov YE. Anaplastic (undifferentiated) carcinoma. In: Nikiforov, Biddinger and Thompson, editors. *Diagnostic Pathology and Molecular Genetics of the Thyroid.* Baltimore, MD: Wolters-Kluwer, LWW; 2009; 228.

[77] Donghi R, Longoni A, Pilotti S, et al. Gene p52 mutations are restricted to poorly differentiated and undifferentiated carcinomas of the thyroid gland. *J. Clin. Invest.,* 1993, 91:179-184.

[78] Garcia-Rostao G, Tallini G, Herraro A, et al. Frequent mutation and nuclear localization of beta-catenin in anaplastic thyroid carcinoma. *Cancer Res.,* 1999, 59:1811-1815.

[79] Garcia-Rostan G; Camp RL; Herrero A; Carcangiu ML; Rimm DL; Tallini G. Beta-catenin dysregulation in thyroid neoplasms: down-regulation, aberrant nuclear expression, and CTNNB1 exon 3 mutations are markers for aggressive tumor phenotypes and poor prognosis. *Am. J. Pathol.,* 2001 Mar, 158(3):987-96.

[80] Santarpia L, El-Naggar AK, Cote GJ, Myers JN, Sherman SI. Phosphatidylinositol 3-inase/Akt and Ras/Raf-mitogen-activated protein kinase pathway mutations in anaplastic thyroid cancer. *J. Clin. Endocrinol. Metab.,* 2008, 93:278–284.

[81] Garcia Rostan G, Zhao H, Camp RL, Pollan M, Talini G et al: Ras mutation are associated with aggressive phenotypes and poor prognosis in anaplastic thyroid cancer. *Journal of Clinical Oncology,* 2003, 21:3226-3235.

[82] Quiros RM, Ding HG, Gattuso P, Prinz et al: Evidence that one subset of anaplastic thyroid carcinomas are derived from papillary carcinomas due to BRAF and p53 mutation. *Cancer,* 2005, 103;2261-2268.

[83] Wiseman SM, Griffith OL, Gown A, Walker B, Jones SJ. Immunophenotyping of thyroid tumors identifies molecular markers altered during transformation of differentiated into anaplastic carcinoma. *Am. J. Surg.,* 2011 May, 201(5):580-6.

[84] Mulligan LM, Kwok JB, Healey CS, et al. Germ-line mutations of the RET proto-oncogene in multiple endocrine neoplasia type 2A. *Nature,* 1993, 363:458-460.

[85] Donis-Keller H, Dou S, chi D, et al. Mutations in the RET proto-oncogene are associated with MEN 2A and FMTC. *Hum. Mol. Genet.,* 1993, 2:851-856.

[86] Eng C, Smith DP, Mulligan LM, et al. Point mutation within the tyrosine kinase domain of the RET proto-oncogene in multiple endocrine neoplasia type 2B and related sporadic tumours. *Hum. Mol. Genet.,* 1994, 3:237-241.

[87] deGroot JW, Links TP, Plukker JT, et al. RET as a diagnostic and therapeutic target in sporadic and hereditary endocrine tumors. *Endocr. Rev.,* 2006, 27:535-560.

[88] Biddinger PW. Medullary Carcinoma. In: Nikiforov, Biddinger and Thompson, editors. *Diagnostic Pathology and Molecular Genetics of the Thyroid.* Baltimore, MD: Wolters-Kluwer, LWW; 2009; 251-254.

[89] DeLellis RA, Lloyd RV, Heitz PU, et al. Pathology and Genetics of Tumours of Endocrine Organs. Lyons: IARC Press; 2004 61A Holm LE, Blomgren H, Lowhagen T. Cancer risks in patients with chronic lymphocytic thyroiditis. *N. Engl. J. Med.,* Mar 7 1985, 312(10):601-4.

[90] Holm LE, Blomgren H, Lowhagen T. Cancer risks in patients with chronic lymphocytic thyroiditis. *N. Engl. J. Med.,* Mar 7 1985, 312(10): 601-4.

[91] Aggarwal N, Swerdlow SH, Kelly LM, et al. Thyroid carcinoma-associated genetic mutations also occur in thyroid lymphomas. *Mod. Pathol.,* 2012, advance online

publication 11 May 2012; doi: 10.1038/ modpathol.2012.73. http://www.nature.com/ modpathol/journal/vaop/ ncurrent/full/modpathol201273a.html.

[92]   Orru G, Coghe F, Gavina F, et al. Rapid multiplex real-time PCR by molecular beacons for different BRAF allele detection in papillary thyroid carcinoma. *Diag. Mol. Pathol.,* 2010, 19(1):1-8.

[93]   Feilchenfeldt J, Totsch M, Sheu SY, et al. Expression of galectin-3 in normal and malignant thyroid tissue by quantitative PCR and immunohistochemistry. *Mod. Pathol.,* 2003, 16(11):1117-1123.

[94]   Savagner F, Rodien P, Reynier P, et al. Analysis of Tg transcripts by real-time TR-PCT in the blood of thyroid cancer patients. *J. Clin. Endocrinol. Metab.,* 2002, 87(2):635-639.

[95]   Kim SW, Lee JI, Kim JW, et al. BRAFV600E mutation analysis in fine-needle aspiration cytology specimens for evaluation of thyroid nodule: A large series in a BRAFV600E-prevalent population. *J. Clin. Endocrinol. Metab.,* 2010, 95:3693-3700.

[96]   Chudova D, Wilde JI, Wang ET, et al. Molecular classification of thyroid nodules using high-dimensionality genomic data. *J. Clin. Endocrinol. Metab.,* 2010, 95:5296-5304.

[97]   Koperek O, Kornauth C, Capper D, et al. Immunohistochemical detection of the BRAF V600E-mutated protein in papillary thyroid carcinoma. *Am. J. Surg. Pathol.,* 2012(June), 36(6):844-850.

[98]   Yemelyanova A, Vang R, Kshirsagar M, et al. Immunohistochemical staining patterns of p53 can serve as a surrogate marker for TP53 mutations in ovarian carcinoma: an immunohistochemical and nucleotide sequencing analysis. *Modern Pathology,* 2011(May), 24: 1248-1253.

[99]   Kocjan G, Chandra A, Cross PA, et al. The interobserver reproducibility of thyroid fine-needle aspiration using the UK Royal College of Pathologists' classification system. *Am. J. Clin. Pathol.,* 2011, 135(6): 852-859.

[100] Crippa S, Dina R. Interobserver reproducibility of thyroid fine-needle aspiration using the UK Royal College of Pathologists' classification system, editorial. *Am. J. Clin. Pathol.,* 2012, 137:833-835.

[101] Salvatore G, Giannini R, Faviana P, et al. Analysis of BRAF point mutation and RET/PTC rearrangement refines the fine-needle aspiration diagnosis of papillary thyroid carcinoma. *J. Clin. Endocrinol. Metab.,* 2004, 89:5175-5180.

[102] Cohen Y, Rosenbaum E, Clark DP, et al. Mutational analysis of BRAF in fine needle aspiration biopsies of the thyroid: a potential application for the preoperative assessment of thyroid nodules. *Clin. Cancer Res.,* 2004, 10:2761-2765.

[103] Riesco-Eizaguirre G, Gutierrez-Martinez P, Garcia-Cabesas MA, et al. The oncogene BRAF V600E is associated with a high risk of recurrence and less differentiated papillary thyroid carcinoma due to the impairment of Na+/I- targeting to the membrane. *Endocr. Relate Cancer,* 2006, 13:257-269.

[104] Sherman SI. Targeted therapy of thyroid cancer. *Brioche Pharmacology,* 2010, 80(5):592-601.

[105] Ohori NP, Nikiforov MN, Schooled KE, et al. Contribution of molecular testing to thyroid fine-needle aspiration cytology of "follicular lesions of undetermined significance/atypia of undetermined significance." *Cancer Cytopathol.,*2010,118:17-23.

[106] Nikiforov YE, Ohori NP, Hodak SP, et al. Impact of mutational testing on the diagnosis and management of patients with cytologically indeterminate thyroid nodules: A prospective analysis of 1056 FNA samples. *J. Clin. Endocrinol. Metab.,* 2011, Aug 96:3390-3397.

[107] Cantara S, Capezzone M, Marchisotta S, et al. Impact of protooncogene mutation detection in cytological specimens from thyroid nodules improves the diagnostic accuracy of cytology. *J. Clin. Endocrinol. Metab.,* 2010 Mar, 95:1365-1369.

[108] Chudova D, Wilde JI, Wang ET, et al. Molecular classification of thyroid nodules using high-dimensionality genomic data. *J. Clin. Endocrinol. Metab.,* 2010 Dec, 95(12):5296-5304. [108A] Alexander EK, Kennedy GC, Baloch ZW et al. Preoperative diagnosis of benign tghyroid nodules with indeterminate cytology. N Engl J Med 2012; 367:705-15. [108B] Mercier ML, D'Haene N, De Neve N et al. Next generation sequencing improves the diagnosis of thyroid FNA specimens with indeterminate cytology. Histopathology, accepted article, doi: 10.1111/his.12461. [108C] Nikiforova MN, Wald AI, Roy S, et al. Targeted next-generation sequencing panel (ThyroSeq) for detection of mutations in thyroid cancer. *J Clin Endocrinol Metab.,* 2013 Nov, 98:1852-1860. [108D]

[109] Haugen BR. Development of a novel molecular classifier to accurately identify benign thyroid nodules in patients with indeterminate FNA cytology (abstract). Paris: *14th International Thyroid Congress,* 15 Sept 2010.

[110] Li H, Robinson KA, Anton B, et al. Cost-effectiveness of a novel molecular test for cytologically indeterminate thyroid nodules. *J. Clin. Endocrinol. Metab.,* 2011, 96:E1719-E1726.

[111] Grogan RH, Mitmaker EJ, Clark OH. The evolution of biomarkers in thyroid cancer—From mass screening to a personalized biosignature. *Cancers,* 2010, 2:885-912.

[112] Saggiorato E, De Pompa R, Volante M, et al. Characterization of thyroid "follicular neoplasms" in fine-needle aspiration cytological specimens using a panel of immunohistochemical markers: a proposal for clinical application. *Endocr. Relat. Cancer,* 2005, 12:305-317.

[113] Raggio E, Camandona M, Solerio D, et al. The diagnostic accuracy of the immunocytochemical markers in the preoperative evaluation of follicular thyroid lesions. *J. Endocrinol. Invest.,* 2010, 33:378-381.

[114] Mineo R, Costantino A, Frasca F, Sciacca L, Russo S, Vigneri R, Belfiore A. activation of the hepatocyte growth factor (HGF)-Met system in papillary thyroid cancer: Biological effects of HGF in thyroid cancer cells depend on Met expression levels. *Endocrinology,* September 1, 2004, 145(9):4355-4365.

[115] Guerriero E, Ferraro A, Desideria D, et al. UbcH10 expression on thyroid fine-needle aspirates. *Cancer Cytopathol.,* 2010,118(3):157-165.

[116] Lappinga PJ, Kip NS, Jin L, et al. HGMA2 gene expression analysis performed on cytologic smears to distinguish benign from malignant thyroid nodules. *Cancer Cytopathol.,* 2010, 118(5):287-297.

[117] Kouniavsky G, Zeiger MA. The quest for diagnostic molecular markers for thyroid nodules with indeterminate or suspicious cytology. *J. Surg. Oncol.,* 2012, 105:438-443.

[118] Griffith OL, Chiu CG, Gown AM, et al. Biomarker panel diagnosis of thyroid cancer: a critical review. *Expert Rev. Anticancer Ther.,* 2008, 132:359-372.

[119] Antonelli A, Fallahi P, Ferrari SM, et al. RET TKI: potential role in thyroid cancers. *Curr. Oncol. Rep.,* 2012, 14:97-104.

[120] Wells SA Jr, Robinson BG, Gagel RF, et al. Vandetanib in patients with locally advanced or metastatic medullary thyroid cancer: a randomized, double-blind phase III trial. *J Clin Oncol.* 2012; 30(2):134.

[121] Sherman S, Differentiated thyroid cancer: Chemotherapy. http://www.uptodate.com/contents/differentiated-thyroid-cancer-chemotherapy?source=related_link, accessed 4 Jun 2014.

In: Horizons in Cancer Research. Volume 55
Editor: Hiroto S. Watanabe

ISBN: 978-1-63463-228-7
© 2015 Nova Science Publishers, Inc.

Chapter 3

The Potential Role of Arsenic Trioxide in the Treatment of Iodine Non-Avid Thyroid Cancer

Eleonore Fröhlich[1,2] and Richard Wahl[1]

[1]Internal Medicine (Dept. of Endocrinology,
Metabolism, Nephrology and Clinical Chemistry),
University of Tuebingen, Tuebingen, Germany
[2]Center for Medical Research, Medical University of Graz,
Graz, Austria

Abstract

Arsenic trioxide (ATO) is an approved second-line medication for acute promyelocytic leukemia (APL). A positive role for this drug in the treatment of solid carcinomas has been proposed but not established yet. According to clinical trials, solid cancers that might benefit from ATO treatment include melanoma, hepatocellular carcinoma, kidney, and hormone-refractory prostate cancers. In combination with other drugs positive effects have been reported for colorectal cancer. Animal models indicated efficacy in glioma or lung cancer and clinical trials have been performed. For thyroid cancer, anti-proliferative, proapoptotic and differentiating effects have been reported.

Toxicity limits the use of ATO as a chemotherapeutic compound. Acute toxic effects during chemotherapy of APL have been described. Another issue in using ATO is its carcinogenicity. As the same mechanisms are involved both in the carcinogenic and therapeutic effects of ATO, it is mainly the dose applied and the cell type exposed to ATO that determines which cellular effect predominates.

For the therapeutic efficacy of ATO, the most relevant effects are cell cycle arrest, induction of apoptosis through the mitochondrial pathway and autophagy. Additional anti-tumor effects include decreased tumor cell migration and invasion. ATO effects are mediated by activation of P3IK/Akt, MAP kinase and NfκB. Differentiating effects caused by ATO include suppression of tumor-relevant proteins such as cell cycle inhibitors, survivin, CD133, metalloproteinases, and upregulation of factors commonly suppressed in tumor cells, such as p53 and Fas. In addition, ATO also induces changes in cellular behaviour, such as decreased tumor cell invasion and increased iodide uptake in thyroid cancer. In the latter, radioiodine treatment of differentiated thyroid cancer is the preferred option after surgery to eliminate residual tumor cells. It is an efficient and selective treatment provided the neoplastic thyrocytes can accumulate iodide. Mutations and over-activity of PI3K/Akt and MAP kinase signalling is crucial in the development and progression of thyroid cancer and serve as targets for differentiating therapy. Differentiation therapy in thyroid cancer aims to restore iodide uptake and thereby increase sensitivity to radioiodine therapy. To achieve this goal a variety of compounds, such as retinoids, inhibitors of tyrosine kinases, of peroxisome proliferator-γ, of DNA methytransferases, and of histone deacetylases are currently being evaluated in clinical trials. None of these single target inhibitors have produced optimal results. It is expected that multi-target compounds and combinations of substances will improve prognosis.

This review introduces arsenic as a toxic and therapeutic agent and illustrates its intracellular metabolism and its cellular targets for its carcinogenic and therapeutic effects. Results of ATO monotherapy and in combination with other compounds in solid cancer cell lines, in tumor xenografts and in clinical trials are reviewed. Based on the existing data, it can be concluded that monotherapy with ATO may not be promising for the treatment of solid cancers but combinations with other therapeutic interventions like ionizing radiation and thermo-therapy with iron oxide nanoparticles and synergism with cytostatic drugs might represent promising treatment options. In view of the specific relationship between the thyroid gland and arsenic, ATO might be a useful agent in the treatment of thyroid cancer.

Introduction

Arsenic occurs in soils, marine sediments and mineral deposits as oxides and sulfides in two biologically important oxidation states, As^{III} and As^{V}. Historically, arsenic has been used as a medicinal agent, a pigment, a pesticide, and an agent with intent to harm (poison). Acute toxicity with inorganic arsenic causes abdominal pain, vomiting and diarrhea, cardiac problems, hemolysis, shock and finally death. The absorption of orally given arsenic is very high and similarly high plasma levels can be achieved by intravenous and oral application [1]. Arsenic in the drinking water at levels higher than 10 µg/l can cause chronic toxicity. In some countries, especially India, Chile, Mexico, Argentina and China, skin lesions, hypertension, ischemia, diabetes, arteriosclerosis, neuropathies and cancer as manifestation for chronic toxicity are observed. An increased incidence of neoplasms after arsenic exposure has been reported for skin, bladder, kidney, liver, prostate and lung. Arsenic has been classified as class I human carcinogen. However, precise mechanisms responsible for its carcinogenicity have not been identified yet, one reason being that animal models fail to reproduce the pathogenic changes in humans.

In contrast to these toxic and carcinogenic effects, arsenic, usually as arsenic trioxide (ATO), is an approved second-line treatment for acute promyelocytic leukemia (APL). Its effects on the thyroid, its cellular targets for carcinogenicity and chemotherapeutic effects are reviewed in the following.

Specific Reaction of Thyroid Metabolism to Arsenic

The interaction of arsenic and thyroid metabolism has been realized for many years. Epidemiological data show that iodine, on the one hand, can reduce the toxicity of arsenic and that, on the other, arsenic acts goitrogenically in regions with low iodine uptake [2]. In Styria in Austria people (arsenic eaters) consumed arsenic as a stimulant at doses generally considered lethal (300-400 mg of white arsenic (arsenic trioxide) or realgar (arsenic trisulfide) each time), but apparently lived long, healthy lives. These people started with low doses of arsenic, typically 10 mg, and slowly increased up to the maximum dosage of 300-400 mg over a period of weeks. The main problem associated with this habit was the high prevalence of goiter and stunted physical and mental growth in children [3]. This effect is due to the action of arsenic as an endocrine disruptor because in normal thyroid glands, arsenic inhibits thyroid hormone production. Inhibition of thyreoperoxidase and/or of type I deiodinase activities are presumed reasons for this effect [4, 5]. Thyroid hormone levels are also involved in the systemic toxicity of arsenic.

In hypothyroidism, induced by thyrostatics, zebrafish and also rats are more susceptible to arsenic poisoning than in the hyperthyroid condition [6, 7]. The increased elimination of arsenic in the urine of hyperthyroid rats may be one of the mechanisms for decreased toxicity [8]. On the other hand, however, when hypothyroidism was induced by exposure of rats to propylthiouracil, protection against hepatotoxicity of arsenic was observed. The authors suspected that increased glutathione levels, which were induced by the propylthiouracil treatment, were responsible for this protection against arsenic toxicity [9]. Later, however, hepatotoxicity was increased, but this might have been due to the hepatotoxic effect of the propylthiouracil. Therefore, arsenic toxicity in chemically-induced hypothyroidism has to be interpreted with caution because of the (hepato)toxicity of the thyrostatics used, i.e. perchlorate and propylthiouracil.

Cellular Effects of Arsenic Compounds

Arsenic compounds are taken up into cells without specific carriers. As^V can substitute phosphate groups, for instance in ATP, but, in general, is much less cytotoxic than As^{III}. Intracellularly As^V is reduced to As^{III} by glyceraldehyde-3-phosphate dehydrogenase, a key enzyme of glycolysis, and purine nucleotide phosphorylase. Glyceraldehyde-3-phosphate dehydrogenase is a major arsenate reductase in erythrocytes, hepatocytes and tumor cells and causes the higher toxicity that arsenic has in these cells. Subsequently, As^{III} is methylated by cytosolic arsenic methyltransferase, which utilizes S-adenosyl methionine as a donor. Methylation of As^{III} interferes with homocysteine transmethylation and folate metabolic recycling (Figure 1).

Methylated arsenic compounds enter cells less readily but possess higher cytotoxicity than inorganic ones. Arsenic uptake and extrusion is different in methylating cells like hepatocytes and non-methylating cells such as urothelial cells and fibroblasts [10]. Whereas methylating cells took up 4% of arsenic after 1 h, non-methylating cells took up 14%.

The latter also accumulated arsenic to a greater extent than methylating cells. Radical formation, by contrast, was 5 times higher in methylating than in non-methylating cells [11]. The mono-, di- and trimethylated and unmethylated As^{III} compounds preferentially react with SH and NH_2 groups. As^{III} forms reactive sulfur-containing molecules with thioredoxin (TRX). The most important role of the TRX system includes redox-signaling, transcriptional regulation, control of intracellular redox status, cell growth defense against oxidative stress and control of apoptosis.

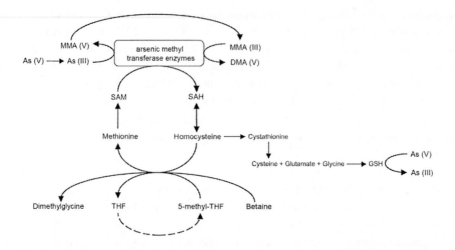

Figure 1. Intracellular metabolism of arsenic compounds. As^V can be reduced to As^{III}, both arsenic compounds can be methylated with one or two methyl groups to monomethylarsenic (MMA) and dimethylarsenic acid/arsenate (DMA). Important cellular metabolites include glutathione (GSH), S-adenosyl methionine (SAM), S-adenosyl homocysteine (SAH) and tetrahydrofolic acid (THF).

The binding of arsenic to thiol groups in cysteine residues and to amino groups in histidine causes loss of function of the respective proteins and appears to be involved in the toxic action of arsenic. Proteins with high affinity for arsenic compounds are poly(ADP-ribose)polymerase, thioredoxin reductase, As(III) methyltransferase, and Kelch-like ECH-associated protein 1 (an interactor with NF-E2-related factor 2, short Nrf2). Nrf2 is a transcription factor that binds to the antioxidant response element of target genes and increases the transcription of a variety of antioxidant and detoxifying enzymes. Reactive oxygen species (ROS) are produced by these interactions, cellular stress responses induced and the detoxification of As^{III} prevented.

Toxicity of Arsenic Compounds

Role of Reactive Oxygen Species (ROS)

ROS signaling pathways can explain most of the cellular effects of arsenic. The generation of ROS is due to the activation of NADPH oxidase and nitric oxide synthase isoenzymes [12], the inhibition of mitochondrial proteins regulating ROS generation, and extracellular export by conjugation to three glutathione molecules. ROS alter protein function by redox reaction with SH-residues [13]. Sulfenic acid (-SOH), sulfinic acid (-SO$_2$H), sulfonic acid (-SO$_3$H) and disulfides (S-S) can be formed. With the exception of sulfonic acid, all reactions are reversible via reducing systems such as thioredoxin and peroxidoxin.

Phosphatidyl Inositol-3 kinase (PI3K)/Akt and Mitogen-Activated Protein (MAP) Kinase Signaling

Phosphatidyl inositol-3 kinases (PI3Ks), particularly class I kinases, are coupled to tyrosine receptor kinases, which are key factors in tumorigenesis (Figure 2). The activated catalytic subunit of PI3K then phosphorylates phosphatidylinositol-4,5-bisphosphate (PIP$_2$) to produce phosphatidylinositol-3,4,5-trisphosphate (PIP$_3$). PIP$_3$ localizes the serine-threonine protein Akt to the cell membrane where Akt becomes phosphorylated and activated by the phosphoinositide-dependent kinases (PDK), most prominently PDK1. An important key negative regulator of this pathway is phosphatase and tensin homolog deleted on chromosome ten (PTEN). PTEN is a phosphatase that dephosphorylates PIP$_3$ and thus terminates signaling of the PI3K/Akt pathway. PTEN itself is inhibited by the proto-oncogene tyrosine-protein kinase SRC.

Phosphorylation of the tyrosine kinase leads to the binding of the cytosolic Growth factor receptor-bound protein 2 (GRB2)/Son of Sevenless (SOS) complex to Ras with subsequent MAP kinase signaling.

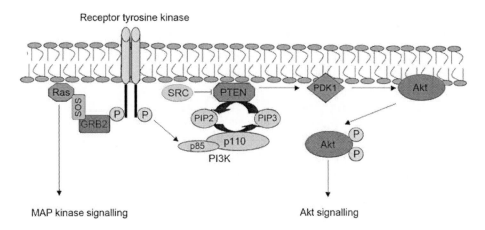

P: phosphate group.

Figure 2. Signaling of receptor tyrosine kinases via activation of the MAP kinase pathway and via the PI3K/Akt pathway. PI3K consists of a p85/p110 heterodimer and catalyses the conversion of phosphatidylinositol-4,5-bisphosphate (PIP$_2$) to phosphatidylinositol-3,4,5-trisphosphate (PIP$_3$). Phosphoinositide-dependent kinase 1 (PDK1) phosphorylates Akt, leading to its activation. The linking of the Growth factor receptor-bound protein 2 (GRB2)/son of sevenless (SOS) complex to Ras starts the MAP kinase signaling cascade. The conversion of PIP$_2$ to PIP$_3$ by phosphatase and tensin homolog deleted on chromosome ten (PTEN) occurs in the close vicinity of the plasma membrane and for all involved proteins association with the membrane has been reported. To include the inhibition of PTEN by the tyrosine kinase protein SRC in the scheme, only the membrane association of PTEN, but not that of PIP$_2$ and PIP$_3$, is shown.

Akt activation regulates cell survival/apoptosis, cell cycle, protein synthesis, and cell growth (Figure 3).

The inhibition of the repressing effect of Glycogen Synthase Kinase-3 (GSK3) on cyclin D1, on p21 and on Myc, stimulation of Mouse Double Minute 2 (MDM2)-induced inhibition of p53 and reduced Forkhead-Related Family of Mammalian Transcription Factor-1 (FKHR) stimulation of p130 and p27 mediate the effects of Akt on the cell cycle.

Cell survival is regulated by inhibition of FKHR/FasL signaling, stimulation of I-kB kinase/Nuclear factor kB (IKK/ NFκB, for its action see Figure 7) and inhibition of apoptosis through reduction of Bcl-XL, caspase 9 and apoptosis signal-regulating kinase 1 (ASK1).

Akt stimulates protein synthesis and cell growth by activation of mammalian target of rapamycin (mTOR), which then stimulates p70 and S6 for increased protein synthesis. mTOR also phosphorylates the pro-apoptotic eukaryotic initiation factor 4E binding protein-1 (4E-BP1) that in its phosphorylated form is prevented from binding to eukaryotic initiation factor 4E (elF-4E). Free elF-4E can bind to the 5'cap of the mRNA transcripts and, through increased translation of cap RNAs, stimulate the synthesis of cell cycle regulators.

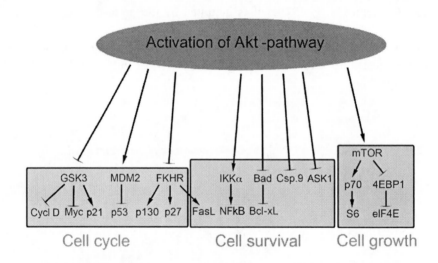

Figure 3. Role of Akt in the cell cycle, survival and cell growth.

Abbreviations: GSK3: Glycogen Synthase Kinase-3; Cycl D: cyclin D; MDM2: Mouse Double Minute 2; FKHR: Forkhead-Related Family of Mammalian Transcription Factor; IKKα: IkB kinase; NfkB: Nuclear factor kappa B; bad: Bcl-2-associated death promoter; Csp. 9: caspase 9; ASK1: apoptosis signal-regulating kinase 1; mTOR: mammalian target of rapamycin; p70: p70 S6 kinase; 4E-BP1: eukaryotic initiation factor 4E binding protein-1; elF-4E: eukaryotic initiation factor 4E.

Mitogen-activated protein (MAP) kinase pathways are of similar importance as PI3K/Akt in tumorigenesis. The kinase cascades of all pathways are organized in a similar way, depicted in Figure 4.

Receptor tyrosine kinases (RTKs), serine/threonine-specific protein kinases, respond to various extracellular signals and modulate physiological reactions and survival of cells. Upon dimerization of RTK, phosphorylation induces the recruitment of the adaptor protein complex GRB2/SOS, which leads to the activation of Ras. Ras acts on→ MEK1/2 and then on→ ERK1/2 which responds predominantly to growth factors and induces proliferation.

Activation of the other MAP kinase cascades is started by specific stimuli (cytokines, hormones, G-protein coupled receptors) or unspecific stimuli such as ROS, UV, heat, pH, metal ions, osmolarity, mechanical stress) which act on a variety of kinases, such as Apoptosis signal-regulating kinase (ASK)1/2, MAP kinase kinase kinase (MKKK, MEKK or MAPKKK)1-4, Thousand-and-one Amino Acid (TAO)1-3, Transforming growth factor (TGF)-β-activated kinase (TAK), Tumor progression locus 2 (Tpl2), mixed lineage kinases (MLK)1-3, dual leucine zipper-bearing kinase (DLK), and leucine-zipper kinase (LZK). MEK3/MEK6 acts on→ p38 α–δ or, alternatively, MKK4/MKK7 activates→ c-Jun NH2-terminal kinase (JNK)1-3/stress activated protein kinase (SAPK) α–γ. This JNK signal transduction pathway transmits the signal to regulate predominantly apoptosis, inflammation and morphogenesis. The role of additional MAP kinase pathways for tumor development, such as the MEK5 → ERK5 cascade and the ERK3K → ERK3 pathway, is less well studied. The ERK5 pathway is of key importance for tumor neovascularization and appears to be a regulator of cell invasion and migration [14]. There is also little information on the role of the ERK3K pathway in cancer; except for participation in tumor cell invasion [15].

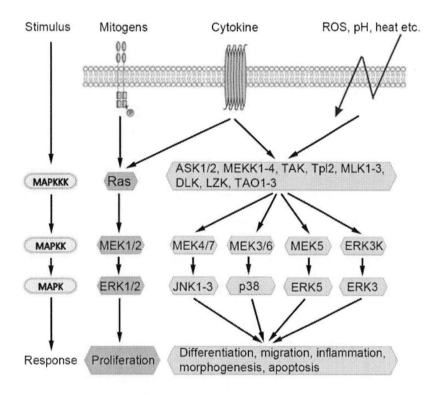

Figure 4. MAP kinase cascades transmit a stimulus to the substrate typically via three kinases. Mitogens, generally, use only the Ras pathway, whereas particularly cytokines may act through all pathways. Abbreviations: ASK: Apoptosis signal-regulating kinase; TAK: Tumor growth factor-β-activated kinase; Tpl2: Tumor progression locus 2; MLK: mixed lineage kinases; DLK: dual leucine zipper-bearing kinase; LZK: leucine-zipper kinase; TAO: Thousand-and-one Amino Acid; Ras: Rat sarcoma; MAPK/MEK: mitogen-activated protein kinase; ERK: extracellular signal-regulated kinase; JNK: c-Jun NH2-terminal kinase.

Dysregulation of PI3K/Akt and MAP kinase pathways is also involved in the development and progression of thyroid cancer (TC).

TC has a much lower incidence (0.74% in men, 2.3% in women worldwide) than cancers of breast, colon, prostate, lung and endometrium but is the seventh most frequent human malignancy and the most common neoplasm of the endocrine system. Carcinoma of follicular origin includes well-differentiated and poorly-differentiated thyroid cancers, and anaplastic thyroid cancers. Differentiated thyroid cancers comprise papillary thyroid carcinoma (PTC), which accounts for 80-90% of all thyroid cancer cases, follicular thyroid carcinoma (FTC) and Hürthle tumors. Undifferentiated/anaplastic thyroid cancer (ATC) is rare and accounts for only 1-2% of all TC. The prognosis of differentiated thyroid cancer is good, with a 10-year survival rate of 85% [16]. Recurrence, however, occurs in up to 30% of patients and only 30% of patients with distant metastases respond to radioiodine therapy with complete remission [17]. A total of 10-20% of the patients develops distant metastases [18]. In this group, the 10-year survival rate drops to 40%. ATC usually has a fatal outcome.

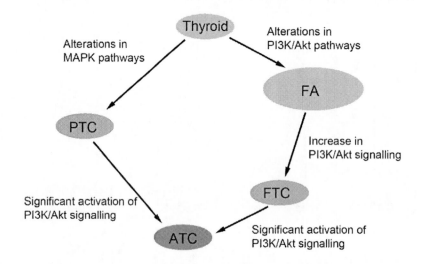

Figure 5. Mutations and overexpression of signaling pathways involved in the development of thyroid cancer. Alterations in MAPK pathways, which lead to papillary thyroid cancer (PTC), include BRAF mutations and RET/PTC rearrangements. Alterations in PI3K/Akt pathways, gene amplifications or mutations, lead to follicular adenoma (FA) with potential development of follicular thyroid cancer (FTC) and anaplastic thyroid cancer (ATC) upon prolonged over-stimulation of the PI3K/Akt pathway.

Alterations of the above-mentioned pathways were linked to the development of the specific histological types of thyroid cancer (Figure 5). Akt kinase expression is increased in sporadic FTC [19]. Mutations in the phosphatidyl inositol-3 kinase catalytic alpha polypeptide (PIK3CA) have been detected at low frequency in follicular thyroid carcinoma (FTC) and anaplastic thyroid carcinoma (ATC). Amplification of PIK3CA, however, has a higher prevalence in thyroid carcinoma and has been identified in 24% and 42% of FTC and ATC, respectively [20, 21]. In general, mutations in PIK3CA and in Akt1 protein appear to be indicators for more aggressive, radioiodine refractory TC [22].

MEK kinase plays an important role in the pathogenesis of TC [23]. Ras mutations in H-, N- and K-Ras oncogenes are common in TC, appear to be an early event in FTC tumorigenesis and are reported in about 50% of FTCs [24]. Tyrosine receptor kinases (TRKs) can activate the MAP pathway through Ras activation and MAPK pathway activation can also augment PI3K signaling. The oncogenic BRAF mutation in the Ras → Raf → MEK → ERK pathway occurs preferentially in PTC, and in some ATC [25]. In PTC, chromosomal inversions and recombinations result in chimeric RET/PTC sequences, which are found in around 30% of TC [26]. RET/PTC is frequently seen in microcarcinoma, suggesting a role in the early phase of tumorigenesis. Increased TRK signaling, evidenced by overexpression of epithelial growth factor receptor expression, is correlated with the presence of metastases in TC [27].

Cellular Targets in the Toxicity of Arsenic Compounds

Intracellular oxidative stress causes genomic aberrations and modification of transcriptional profiles, in addition to single- and double strand breaks. Epigenetic changes are mostly caused by methylated arsenic methylarsonous acid and include changes in DNA methylation, in histone maintenance and in miRNA expression [28, 29]. DNA damage is caused by oxidation in methylating cells. In cells with high and low conversion of arsenic, epigenetic changes such as hypo- and hypermethylation of the DNA have been described.

Mitochondria are another main target for arsenic cytotoxicity. TRX2, TRX peroxidase, glutaredoxin family members, Factor B, all possessing vicinal reactive SH-groups, are localized in mitochondria and inactivated by As^{III}. The binding of As^{III} to voltage-dependent anion channels of the outer membrane and the adenine nucleotide transporter of the inner membrane is linked to the increased permeability of the mitochondrial membrane.

Arsenic also influences autophagy. The role of autophagy in cancer is currently not clear: it protects tumor cells deprived of nutrients but may also act tumorigenically [30]. It is assumed that in normal cells autophagy protects against transformation [31] because PI3K/Akt activation, Bcl-2 amplification, loss of function of PTEN and TP53 and monoallelic loss of Beclin-1 all inhibit autophagy. In tumors, autophagy supports tumor growth and progression. Arsenic can induce autophagy by ERK1/2 signaling and Death-associated protein kinase promotor hypermethylation in urothelial cells [32, 33], thus promoting transformation.

In neuronal SH-SY5Y cells, low concentrations of ATO induce proliferation by ERK1/2 activation and vascular endothelial growth factor (VEGF) secretion [34].

Chemotherapeutic Use of Arsenic

Arsenic compounds have been used for decades for medical purposes in the form of external creams, oral preparations, and injections. In Traditional Chinese medicine, often considered alternative or complementary medicine, arsenic compounds are used as antiseptic agents or in the treatment of rheumatoid diseases, syphilis and psoriasis. In the western world, the arsenic-containing Fowler's solution of potassium arsenite was employed to treat eczema, asthma and psoriasis. Already in the first century AD, arsenic trioxide (ATO) was suggested for the treatment of solid tumors. During the 18th and 19th centuries, ATO represented the main treatment for leukemia but in the 20th century other chemotherapies with less chronic toxicity than arsenic replaced treatment with ATO. Only in China, patients suffering from leukemia were still treated with ATO and the exceptional effect of ATO in a small cohort of patients with a specific type of leukemia, APL, was identified. Long-lasting remissions of APL patients upon treatment with ATO were reproduced later in larger cohorts and finally led to the approval of ATO, commercially distributed as Trisenox®, as second-line treatment for APL.

ATO induces apoptosis, possesses antiproliferative activity and inhibits angiogenesis in APL [35]. Mechanisms involved in the chemotherapeutic effect of ATO in APL include induction of apoptosis by elevated H_2O_2 levels, cytochrome release and caspase activation, increased bax expression, inhibition of the NfκB pathway, inhibition of GTP-induced polymerization of tubulin, and altered nuclear distribution of promyelocytic leukemia protein (PML). Inhibition of Signal transducer and activator of transcription 3 (STAT3) activity, growth arrest in the G1 phase and induction of differentiation were related to the antiproliferative activity of ATO. Angiogenesis was inhibited via the decreased expression of VEGF.

In contrast to its established role in APL and promising results in other hematological malignancies, the role of ATO in solid carcinomas is not yet established. The screening of cell lines derived from solid carcinomas performed by Yang et al. [36] identified bladder carcinoma and gastrointestinal carcinomas as sensitive cell lines. Clinical trials with patients suffering from these carcinomas, however, were not successful [37-40] and only modest effects were observed in pancreatic cancer [41], advanced melanoma [42] and refractory colon cancer [43]. On the other hand, Phase II trials in hormone-refractory prostate cancers confirmed the cytostatic effect [44], which had been seen in xenograft models in animals [37]. Other clinical trials have been completed but data are not analyzed yet. Table I presents an overview on trial results and completed trials with ATO as monotherapy or in combination with other interventions in solid carcinomas.

Animal studies showed antitumor effects in orthotopic models for androgen-independent prostate cancer, breast cancer, hepatoma and glioma [37, 57-60] and also in xenograft models of lung carcinoma and nasopharyngeal carcinoma [61-63]. In addition, ATO suppressed invasion of intraperitoneally-injected ovarian carcinoma cells [64] and induced apoptosis in xenografts of gastric cancer cells [65]. The formation of metastases upon iv injection of hepatoma cells [66] was also suppressed by ATO. In studies with xenografts of Ewing sarcoma, however, less positive results were obtained [67].

Efficiency of ATO in vitro was also seen in cell lines of bladder, colon, lung, renal, cervix, thyroid and gastric cancer [68, 69]. There is still the hope that improved pharmaceutical applications, e.g. inclusion in nanoparticles and improved targeting, will improve the efficacy of ATO. Liposomal encapsulated ATO and folate-targeted ATO-loaded liposomes have shown promising results in vitro and in vivo and may go to pre-clinical testing [57, 70]. The synthetic tripeptide arsenical para-4 [N(S-glutathionylacetyl)amino] phenyl arsenoxide (GSAO), one of the few arsenic-based antineoplastic compounds other than ATO, acts especially on mitochondrial pores. This compound blocks the adenine nucleotide transporter in an open position, thereby causing an increase in superoxide radicals, depolarization of mitochondria, and decreased proliferation and apoptosis of endothelial cells. In tumor xenografts the compound decreases angiogenesis [71].

Table 1. Results of clinical trials on ATO in solid carcinomas

Phase	Description	Status	Ref.
I	ATO, Astrocytoma in childhood, 21 patients	Result: safe dose confirmed	[45]
I	ATO + temozolomide + radiation, glioma, 17 patients	Result: well tolerated, 1 CR, 5 PR	[46]
I	ATO + radiation, newly diagnosed glioma	Trial completed	RNP
I	ATO + radiation, glioma	Trial completed	RNP
I	ATO + temozolomide + radiation, glioma	Trial completed	RNP
I	ATO + radiosurgery, recurrent malignant glioma	Trial completed	RNP
I	ATO, Stage IV melanoma, 17 patients	Result: 10 SD	[47]
I	ATO + radiation + hyperthermia, head and neck cancer, 11 patients	Result: safe dose confirmed	[48]
I	ATO + 5-FU + Leucovorin, refractory colorectal carcinoma, 12 patients	Result: safe dose confirmed	[49]
I	ATO + 5-FU + Leucovorin, colorectal carcinoma	Trial completed	RNP
Pilot	ATO + ascorbic acid, metastatic colorectal carcinoma, 5 patients	Result: no CR or PR	[43]
II off	ATO, metastatic colorectal carcinoma, 6 patients	Result: 2 PR, 4 SD	[50]
II	ATO, primary hepatocellular carcinoma, 102 patients	Result: pain reduction, 7 PR, 71 SD	[51]
II	ATO, hepatocellular carcinoma, 29 patients	Result: 1 PR, 3 SD	[52]
II	ATO, non resectable hepatocellular carcinoma	Trial completed	RNP
II	ATO, pancreatic carcinoma, refractory to gemcitabine, 13 patients	Result: no objective responses	[41]
II	ATO, pancreatic carcinoma, refractory to gemcitabine	Trial completed	RNP
II	ATO, metastatic kidney cancer, 14 patients	Result: 3 SD	[39]
II	ATO, metastatic kidney cancer	Trial completed	RNP
II	ATO, recurrent urothelial carcinoma, 12 patients	Result: 4 SD	[53]
II	ATO, urothelial carcinoma	Trial completed	RNP
II	ATO, Refractory germ cell cancer, 20 patients	Result: no CR or PR	[54]
II	ATO, hormone-refractory prostate carcinoma, 19 patients	Result: no CR or PR; 2 decrease of PSA	[44]
II	ATO, hormone-refractory prostate carcinoma	Trial completed	RNP
Pilot	ATO + radiation, breast cancer, 7 patients	Result: 3 CR, 3 PR, 1 SD	[55]
II	ATO, metastatic breast carcinoma	Trial completed	RNP
II	ATO, cervical cancer IVB	Trial completed	RNP
II	ATO, metastatic melanoma, 20 patients	Result: no CR, 8 SD	[56]
II	ATO + ascorbic acid + temozolomide, metastatic melanoma, 40 patients	Result: no objective responses	[42]
II	Advanced metastatic non-small cell lung cancer	Trial completed	RNP

PR: partial response; SD: stable disease; RNP: results not yet published, *: off protocol

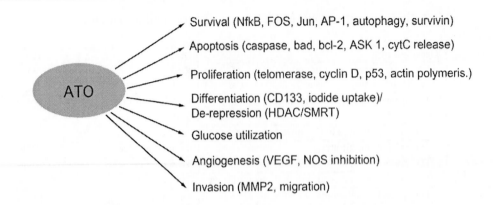

Figure 6. ATO acts by various mechanisms on cell survival/apoptosis, on proliferation and on differentiation. Typical tumor properties like increased glucose utilization, angiogenesis and invasion are additional targets for the multi-targeted action of ATO.

The main modes of ATO action in solid cancer cell lines were similar to those identified for hematological malignancies and are summarized in Figure 6.

Role of PI3K/Akt and MAPK Signaling in the Cytostatic Effect of ATO

Effects on MAPK pathways differed between cancer types. Thus, in mesothelioma ATO acted on the JNK pathway [72]. In cervix cancer [73], lung cancer [74], melanoma and hepatoma effects were mediated by MAP kinase [75] signaling. ATO stimulated the ERK pathway in retinoblastoma and osteosarcoma [76, 77]. Activation of JNK was also seen in normal hepatocytes, although at higher concentrations of 20-40 µM [78].

Nrf2 regulation transmitted the effect of ATO in squamous oral carcinoma and glioma [79, 80]. Of note, the effect of ATO on Nrf2 differed between in-vitro and in-vivo observations; ATO activated the pathway in oral squamous carcinoma cells in-vitro but down-regulated it in-vivo.

Cellular Targets for the Cytostatic Effect of ATO

Transcription was influenced by reversal of epigenetic changes, namely by inhibition of DNA-methyltransferase and of histone deacetylase, and by inhibition of telomerase in breast cancer, cervix cancer, endometrial cancer, colon cancer and pancreas cancer cell lines [81-83].

Mitochondria were identified as the main targets of ATO effects in uveal melanoma [84], colon cancer, urothelial bladder cancer, prostate cancer, pancreatic cancer, gastric cancer, oral squamous carcinoma, hepatoma and lung cancer [85-88]. Changes in mitochondrial metabolism include decreased mitochondrial membrane potential and induction of the mitochondrial pathway of apoptosis.

Induction of autophagy was involved in the cytostatic effect of ATO in ovarian cancer and glioblastoma [89]. However, it has also been implicated as a mechanism of carcinogenesis in uroepithelial cells [33]. The fact that induction of autophagy was involved in both carcinogenic and chemotherapeutic actions is consistent with the dual role of increased autophagy as an inhibitor of tumorigenesis in normal cells and promoter of tumor growth in established tumors [31].

ATO induces apoptosis in retinoblastoma [76, 90], uveal melanoma [84], lung cancer [85], gastric cancer, cholangiocarcinoma [91], hepatoma [92, 93], colorectal cancer [94], squamous carcinoma [88], cervix cancer [95], endometrial cancer [82], prostate cancer [86], urothelial bladder cancer [86] and osteosarcoma [96], acting via different mechanisms. In normal fibroblasts, the mitochondrial membrane potential decreased, Bcl-2 decreased and caspase 8 increased, which also led to apoptosis, but these cells were more resistant to ATO than transformed cells [68].

Induction of cell cycle arrest, inhibition of neo-angiogenesis and decreased migration were important mechanisms of action identified in cervix cancer [95, 97], lung cancer [98], gastric cancer [99, 100], gall bladder cancer [101], Ewing sarcoma [102] and osteosarcoma [77, 103] cell lines under ATO treatment.

Increased cellular differentiation was either caused by the decrease of cancer stem cells or by the re-appearance of physiological reactions in thyroid cancer [69] and breast cancer [104, 105]. In gynecological cancers, the re-expression of estrogen receptor alpha could be used for re-sensitization to endocrine therapy such as tamoxifen [104]. On the other hand, ATO can suppress growth of estrogen-dependent tumors by decreasing estrogen receptor-alpha expression and estrogen-dependent signaling in breast carcinoma cell lines [106, 107] and in endometrial cancer cells [108].

Cancer stem cells play a great role in the resistance of tumor to chemotherapy and novel approaches aim to induce re-differentiation in these cells. ATO induced apoptosis specifically in CD133$^+$ gall bladder carcinoma stem cells [101] and by down-regulation of the stem cell marker Sox2 in glioma cells [109]. Down-regulation of Gli1, the transcription factor involved in sonic hedgehog signaling of cancer stem cells, increased tumor differentiation and induced prolonged survival of mice with hepatocellular carcinoma xenografts [110]. Binding of ATO to Gli1 also increased the efficacy of chemostatic drugs, such as gemcitabine in pancreatic cancer cells [111]. ATO in combination with metformin promoted autophagy and differentiation in glioma by decrease of CD133$^+$ cells [112].

Co-Treatment with ATO

As most effects of ATO appear to be caused by ROS generation, it was combined with oxidants (buthionine sulfoximine, ascorbic acid) in several cells and seems to have shown increased efficacy. Combined with other drugs, radiation or hyperthermia, increased efficacy compared to monotherapy was observed, via action on the main target and/or action on an additional target. ATO has been combined with conventional chemotherapeutic treatments (e.g. cisplatin, paclitaxel, 5-fluouracil, ionizing radiation, hyperthermia), with differentiating drugs (tyrosine kinase inhibitors, histone deacetylase inhibitors), non-steroidal antiphlogistic drugs (sulindac), and other organic, not yet established chemotherapeutics (e.g. oridonin, silibinin, humeic acid). The advantage of dual therapy including ATO was tumor and combination-specific. Upon co-treatment with ATO, improved efficacy and responses in resistant tumor cells were obtained; for other tumors, a reduction of the cytostatic agent could be achieved. Dose reductions of chemostatic drugs are advantageous because they are accompanied by a reduced incidence of adverse effects.

One advantage of the combined treatment of cervix cancer cells with ATO plus oxidants was its improved efficacy independent of the glutathione levels [113].

In combination with chemotherapeutic drugs like cisplatin, ATO induced apoptosis in urothelial bladder cells [114], in lung cancer cells [115] and in glioblastoma cells [116] to a higher extent than when used alone. In ovarian cancer cells this combination allowed a reduction in the dose of cisplatin [117]. In addition to cisplatin, the drug-sensitizing effect of ATO was also observed on co-application with the alkylating drug 3a-aza-cyclopenta[a]indene in urothelial bladder cells [118], with paclitaxel in several cell lines [119] and together with doxorubicin, Interferon $-\alpha 2b$, capecitabine in hepatoma cells [120]. In glioblastoma, synergistic effects were observed by combining ATO with ionizing radiation plus the alkyating agent temozolomide and the humanized anti-VEGF antibody bevacizumab [121]. The nucleobase 5-Fluorouracil together with ATO decreased proliferation by inhibition of thymidilate synthase in colorectal carcinoma [122]. The combination of ATO + rapamycin takes advantage of the interaction between mTOR and Akt pathways (Figure 3). In this combination ATO attenuated Akt pathway activation by rapamycin in breast cancer cells [123].

Synergistic effects were also observed with differentiating drugs such as the histone deacetylase inhibitor Suberoylanilide Hydroxamic Acid in lung cancer cells [124] and with the tyrosine kinase inhibitor sorafenib in hepatoma cells [125]. Retinoic acid increased the effect of ATO in U87MG glioma cells with p53 codon-specific hot spot mutation grown as neurospheres [126].

In combination with the nucleoside analogue, 3-azido-3-deoxythymidine, telomerase inhibition and apoptosis were increased in xenografts from gastric cancer cells [127]. The combination with the immunostimulatory ds RNA analogue Polyinosinic:polycytidylic acid was effective in gastric cancer cells by increasing mitochondrial dysfunction and apoptosis [128].

The combination of ATO with other drugs, such as the sesquiterpene lactone parthenolide and the non-steroidal anti-inflammatory drug sulindac, increased apoptosis in xenografts from pancreatic [129] and lung cancer cells, respectively [130]. Different mechanisms were reported for the synergism with sulindac in lung and colon cancer cells, either by activation of the MAPK pathway, by JNK or by degradation of the NfκB inhibitor IKb [130-132]. The combination of ganciclovir and ATO synergistically induced apoptosis in nasopharyngeal cancer cells [133].

The synergism with drugs from Traditional Chinese Medicine such as the alkaloid berberine in glioblastoma was mediated through a variety of mechanisms, namely increased apoptosis, decreased metalloproteinase expression, and cytoskeletal rearrangement [134, 135]. Oridonin + ATO increased apoptosis in a hepatoma mouse model [136].

Compounds with unclear antitumor action, such as the flavonoid silibinin and the organic degradation polymer humic/fluvic acid, increased efficacy of ATO in glioblastoma cells and cervical cancer cells, respectively [137, 138]. Humic acid often coexists with arsenic in water and, at low concentrations, could promote tumor progression; at high concentrations, reduced viability in lung cancer cells was observed [139]. In co-treatment with humic acid plus ATO, an increased pro-apoptotic effect was particularly noticeable. Interestingly, the chemostatic and carcinogenic action of this combination was also mediated through the same molecular and cellular targets, signaling by PI3K/Akt, MAPK and NfκB, migration, adhesion and invasion. Similarly, Icariin increased the efficacy of ATO in hepatocellular carcinoma xenografts by induction of ROS generation via decreased NfκB activity [140].

Combined with ionizing radiation (external beam radiation), ATO killed osteosarcoma cells more efficiently than radiation alone through Akt signaling [141] and in prostate cancer cells through Akt/mTOR signaling [142]. In fibrosarcoma xenografts, tumor growth reduction via ERK1/2 activation and increased autophagy has been reported [141]. Similar mechanisms also triggered greater efficacy in glioma cells [143]. In cervix carcinoma cells, ATO + ionizing radiation caused activation of MAPK and JNK pathways [73]. Another group identified activation of apoptosis as the main mechanism in cervix carcinoma cells [38]. The optimum effect was obtained in osteosarcoma xenografts because efficacy was increased while side effects, such as loss of normal bone, were reduced [144].

In tumor models, additional effects of the synergistic action of ATO and radiation have been identified: ATO was able to shut down tumor vasculature, and, thereby, reduced the size of fibrosarcoma in mice [145]. The radiosensitizing effect of ATO was also seen in glioma, cervical and head and neck squamous carcinoma [146]. In other murine tumor studies it is hypothesized that ATO inhibits mitochondrial respiration and increases sensitivity to radiation by increasing tumor oxygenation via a decrease in oxygen consumption [147].

The combination of ATO plus physical treatment (hyperthermia) with iron oxide nanoparticles reduced tumor growth of cervix cancer, hepatoma and fibrosarcoma xenografts and in the rabbit liver tumor model VX2 [104, 148-150]. The observed effects were elicited both by apoptosis and by vascular shut down.

Problems in the Therapeutic Use of ATO

Despite promising in-vitro results and greater efficacy of several drugs upon co-application, the use of ATO as a chemotherapeutic drug presents several problems. The acute toxicity of arsenic compounds is high and cardiovascular problems in patients under medication with ATO for APL have been reported [151]. Secondly, sensitivity to ATO showed prominent differences between line lines. IC_{50} values of ATO in the breast cancer cell line MCF-7 and the ovarian cancer line A2780 were 4 - 5 times lower than in the lung cancer cell lines H520, H322 and H460 [152]. At a concentration of 20 μM ATO 80% of HeLa cells were apoptotic, whereas the fraction of apoptotic cells in the A549 cell line was only 10% [153]. It is likely that also the mode of action differed between the primary endothelial cells, and cell lines from endothelia, lung cancer and cervix cancer. In some cell lines a tight correlation of reactive oxygen species and loss of mitochondrial membrane potential to the apoptotic effect was identified, whereas in others no link between radical stress and apoptosis was seen [153].

Thirdly, the action of ATO was dose-dependent. Proliferation of colon cancer cells increased at low ATO concentrations and decreased at higher concentrations [154]. Similarly, high (>10μM) concentrations of ATO inhibited NfκB, low and non-cytotoxic concentrations activated this transcription factor in mouse epidermal cells [155]. NfκB activates the cyclin D1 promotor (Figure 7) and high cyclin D1 levels are required for progression of the cells into the S-phase. Low ATO levels, consequently, promote tumorigenesis whereas high levels induce cell cycle arrest.

The dose-dependency of the effect is undesired because normal cells, such as fibroblasts, are more resistant to ATO toxicity than transformed cells. Unfortunately, with concentrations used for therapy (1-5 μM ATO) proliferation in these cells is increased [68].

There are currently no data available that show if ATO treatment in APL increases long-term complications as observed with environmental exposure to arsenic derivatives, in particular an increased incidence of malignancies.

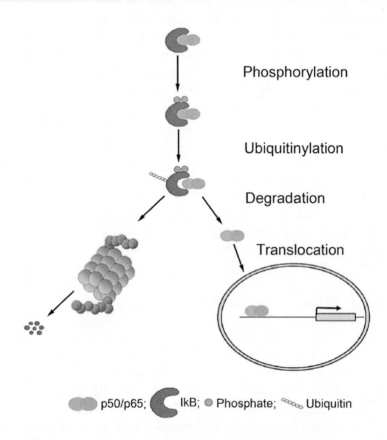

Figure 7. Action of NfκB on transcription of DNA. NfκB (p50/p65 heterodimer) is located in the cytoplasm in complexes with its inhibitor IkB. Activation of NfκB starts with the activation of IkB kinase for phosphorylation of IkB. This induces ubiquitinylation and subsequent degradation of IkB in the proteasome. After degradation of its inhibitor, NfκB translocates into the nucleus and binds to the promoter region of NfκB target genes, such as cyclin D1, c-myc, Bcl-xL, p21/cip1, relB, and others.

ATO in Thyroid Cancer Treatment

Standard treatment of well-differentiated TC is surgery followed by radioiodine (RAI) remnant ablation. As only thyrocytes take up iodide to a large degree, radioiodine treatment is very specific and has a low rate of adverse effects. For ATCs, which neither take up iodide nor produce thyroglobulin, surgical resection is only recommended for localized disease. At the advanced stage, patients do not profit from removal of the tumor mass. Palliation to improve survival includes tracheotomy, radiation and chemotherapy and combinations of these.

At least 30% of patients with differentiated thyroid carcinoma show insufficient iodide uptake [156], caused by transcriptional and post-translational changes in sodium-/iodide transporter (NIS) expression. In cases of insufficient iodine uptake, treatment options are limited and prognosis poor. External beam radiation is used as palliative therapeutic option but these tumors are usually unresponsive to this therapy. Adriamycin (doxorubicin) is the only cytostatic drug approved by the FDA for treatment of radioiodine refractory thyroid carcinoma.

Targeted Therapies for TC

Targeted therapies have the potential to reverse the pathological changes that led to tumor formation through the inhibition of up-regulated pathways.

Tyrosine kinase inhibitors, such as sunitinib (Sutent®), pazopanib (Votrient®), and axitinib (Inlyta®) act mainly by inhibition of VEGF signalling, while thalidomide (Contergan®) and lenalidomide (Revlimid® act by a variety of poorly understood mechanisms independent of VEGF signalling. Many of these inhibitors showed promising results in preclinical models but performed less well in the clinic. For more information on the status of tyrosine kinase inhibitors in clinical trials the reader is referred to one of the more extensive reviews on this topic [157, 158]. A phase III trial for sorafenib in locally advanced or metastatic RAI-refractory DTC (NCT00984282) was initiated [159]. In this trial partial responses of 12% were obtained [160].

The authors explained the limited success of the drug by the fact that EGFR inhibitors, including Iressa® (Gefitinib, ZD1939), are ineffective in tumors with Raf mutations. The BRAF inhibitor Sorafenib (BAY 43-9006) achieved partial responses and stable disease in patients with radioiodine-refractory thyroid cancer. XL281, a pan-RAF inhibitor, induced stable disease in PTC patients. PLX 4032 (RG7204, RO5185426, Vemurafenib) inhibits only mutated BRAF, mediating prolonged stable disease in a small phase I study. AZD6244 (ARRY142886, Selumetinib), a MEK1 and MEK2 inhibitor, showed similar efficacy, when used in monotherapy 3% [161]. While these trials assessed single agent efficacy, TK inhibitors might be more effective in combination with RAI treatment. The combination of selumetinib with RAI treatment in the study by Ho et al. [162] reported partial responses of 63% in patients with DTC (overall rate was 25%). This high rate of partial responses was mainly due to strict patient selection for RAI treatment.

Differentiating drugs are expected to re-induce differentiation by reversal of the pathogenetic cell alterations. Epigenetic changes, namely increased histone deacetylation and methylation of DNA, play an important role in the development of thyroid cancer because these changes silence genes involved in the differentiation of thyrocytes. In a phase II trial with the histone deacetylase inhibitor SAHA, approved by the FDA as Zolinza®, slightly more patients with stable disease than with progressive disease were reported [163]. In a phase II study, romidepsin, a depsipeptide with the tradename Istodax (FK 228, FR 901228) restored radioiodine avidity in 2 of the 20 patients treated, but there were no objective responses even after ^{131}I treatment [164]. A phase II study on the new hydroxamic acid-derived non-selective histone deacetylase inhibitor panbinostat (LBH589) is currently recruiting participants. The recruitment status of a phase II study on Depakene® (valproic acid) initiated in 2007, is unknown (http://www.clinicaltrials.gov). A phase II trial on Vidaza® (5-azacytidine), a DNA methyltransferase inhibitor, in metastatic TC has been completed and results will be published soon. A phase II study on Decitabine® (5-Aza-2'-deoxycytidine) is listed as an ongoing clinical trial evaluating re-differentiation for TC (http://www.clinicaltrials.gov).

Retinoic acid and the peroxisome proliferator activated receptor-γ agonist rosiglitazone increased radioiodine uptake to variable degree in phase II trials [165-170]. Efficacy and problems in the assessment of these compounds have been reviewed recently [171].

Additional compounds resulting in stable disease in clinical trials target the cytoskeleton and the proteasome. The prodrug Combre(ta)statin A4 phosphate binds to tubulin and destabilizes tumor blood vessels. In a trial with ATC the compound induced stable disease in 30% of the patients. Meta-analysis in a phase II trial on Velcade® (bortezomib) achieved mainly stable disease in metastasized differentiated thyroid cancer.

These data show that a variety of drugs are in various phases of pre-clinical evaluation for the treatment of thyroid cancer and that therapeutic options are still suboptimal.

Radiation Treatment in TC

Remnant ablation therapy with RAI and external beam radiation treatment (EBRT) are established therapies for TC. According to the guidelines of the American Thyroid Association (ATA), RAI is recommended for metastatic disease, primary tumors > 4 cm and tumors 1-4 cm with lymph node metastases. EBRT is indicated for patients older than 45 years with gross residual non-radioiodine-avid tumors and for palliation of individual metastatic lesions such as brain metastases and possibly lung metastases [172]. It is suggested that metastatic TC of all histology, especially brain metastases, profit from EBRT [173]. RAI acts as a cytotoxic agent either by causing apoptosis or necrosis, depending on the dose. Studies in the differentiated thyroid carcinoma cell line B-CPAP indicated that ^{131}I-radioactivity below 10 MBq/ml mainly induced apoptosis, whereas at doses > 10 MBq/ml necrosis predominated [174]. Cell death caused by EBRT appears to be mediated mostly either by apoptosis or by mitotic catastrophe. Less often necrosis, cellular senescence and autophagy are involved [175]. More recently, another mechanism, necroptosis, or programmed necrosis, has been reported in radiation-induced cell death of ATC [176].

Effect of ATO in TC Cell Lines

Pharmacological concentrations (2 μM) of ATO result in reduced proliferation and increased apoptosis and iodide uptake in various differentiated thyroid cancer cell lines [69]. Protein levels of NIS and pendrin (PDS) were not changed but in ATO-treated cells PDS displayed a polarized expression pattern. Depletion of glutathione increased the differentiating effect of ATO while Akt-inhibitors did not. Independent of the proliferation rate, ATO significantly decreased glucose uptake in TC cells as one additional mechanism of its multi-modal action.

Conclusion

Based on its efficacy in studies with thyroid cancer cell lines, the multi-target action of ATO appears suited for the therapy of RAI-resistant differentiated thyroid cancers. For other malignancies, promising clinical trials are already available. ATO can be combined with other antineoplastic drugs for improved efficacy. The combination of radiation together with ATO treatment could be helpful not only for the therapy of differentiated but also for anaplastic thyroid carcinoma. Therapies with cisplatin, doxorubicin or docetaxel and EBRT are effective but have severe adverse effects. Based on in-vivo-studies with several solid cancers it is expected that the combination of radiation and ATO-assisted treatment is less toxic and, therefore, could be an option for palliative radiation treatment in TC. The carcinogenic effects of ATO on normal cells are not yet clarified because no data on long-term effects in patients treated with ATO in APL are available so far. In any case, duration of treatment may be too short for ATO to exert carcinogenic effects. It is also currently unclear to which extent thyroid hormone status and interactions between iodide metabolism and arsenic, reported in the section 'Specific reaction of thyroid metabolism and arsenic', can influence the therapeutic effect of ATO. Such influences could be relevant because patients are usually subjected either to thyroid hormone withdrawal or to stimulation with thyroid stimulating hormone prior to RAI treatment.

References

[1] Kumana CR, Au WY, Lee NS, Kou M, Mak RW, Lam CW, et al. Systemic availability of arsenic from oral arsenic-trioxide used to treat patients with hematological malignancies. *Eur J Clin Pharmacol*. 2002; 58 (8): 521-526.

[2] Sharpless G, Metzger M. Arsenic and goiter. *J Nutr*. 1940; 21 341-346.

[3] Emsley J (2006) *"Arsenic". The Elements of Murder: A History of Poison*. Ed. (Oxford University Press, Oxford).

[4] Davey JC, Nomikos AP, Wungjiranirun M, Sherman JR, Ingram L, Batki C, et al. Arsenic as an endocrine disruptor: arsenic disrupts retinoic acid receptor-and thyroid hormone receptor-mediated gene regulation and thyroid hormone-mediated amphibian tail metamorphosis. *Environ Health Perspect*. 2008; 116 (2): 165-172.

[5] Palazzolo DL, Jansen KP. The minimal arsenic concentration required to inhibit the activity of thyroid peroxidase activity in vitro. *Biol Trace Elem Res*. 2008; 126 (1-3): 49-55.

[6] Allen T, Rana SV. Oxidative stress by inorganic arsenic: modulation by thyroid hormones in rat. *Comp Biochem Physiol C Toxicol Pharmacol*. 2003; 135 (2): 157-162.

[7] Liu F, Gentles A, Theodorakis CW. Arsenate and perchlorate toxicity, growth effects, and thyroid histopathology in hypothyroid zebrafish Danio rerio. *Chemosphere*. 2008; 71 (7): 1369-1376.

[8]   Rana SV, Allen T. Influence of thyroxine and n-propylthiouracil on nephro-toxicity of inorganic arsenic in rat. *Toxicol Ind Health*. 2006; 22 (3): 137-145.

[9]   Allen T, Rana SV. Effect of n-propylthiouracil or thyroxine on arsenic trioxide toxicity in the liver of rat. *J Trace Elem Med Biol*. 2007; 21 (3): 194-203.

[10]   Dopp E, von Recklinghausen U, Diaz-Bone R, Hirner AV, Rettenmeier AW. Cellular uptake, subcellular distribution and toxicity of arsenic compounds in methylating and non-methylating cells. *Environ Res*. 2010; 110 (5): 435-442.

[11]   Dopp E, von Recklinghausen U, Hartmann LM, Stueckradt I, Pollok I, Rabieh S, et al. Subcellular distribution of inorganic and methylated arsenic compounds in human urothelial cells and human hepatocytes. *Drug Metab Dispos*. 2008; 36 (5): 971-979.

[12]   Rao J. The other side of arsenic. *Al Ameen J Med Sci*. 2009; 2 (Special): 51-56.

[13]   Ray PD, Huang BW, Tsuji Y. Reactive oxygen species (ROS) homeostasis and redox regulation in cellular signaling. *Cell Signal*. 2012; 24 (5): 981-990.

[14]   Lochhead PA, Gilley R, Cook SJ. ERK5 and its role in tumour development. *Biochem Soc Trans*. 2012; 40 (1): 251-256.

[15]   Long W, Foulds CE, Qin J, Liu J, Ding C, Lonard DM, et al. ERK3 signals through SRC-3 coactivator to promote human lung cancer cell invasion. *J Clin Invest*. 2012; 122 (5): 1869-1880.

[16]   Eustatia-Rutten CF, Corssmit EP, Biermasz NR, Pereira AM, Romijn JA, Smit JW. Survival and death causes in differentiated thyroid carcinoma. *J Clin Endocrinol Metab*. 2006; 91 (1): 313-319.

[17]   Dohan O, De la Vieja A, Paroder V, Riedel C, Artani M, Reed M, et al. The sodium/iodide Symporter (NIS): characterization, regulation, and medical significance. *Endocr Rev*. 2003; 24 (1): 48-77.

[18]   Durante C, Haddy N, Baudin E, Leboulleux S, Hartl D, Travagli JP, et al. Long-term outcome of 444 patients with distant metastases from papillary and follicular thyroid carcinoma: benefits and limits of radioiodine therapy. *J Clin Endocrinol Metab*. 2006; 91 (8): 2892-2899.

[19]   Ringel MD, Hayre N, Saito J, Saunier B, Schuppert F, Burch H, et al. Overexpression and overactivation of Akt in thyroid carcinoma. *Cancer Res*. 2001; 61 (16): 6105-6111.

[20]   Liu D, Mambo E, Ladenson PW, Xing M. Letter re: uncommon mutation but common amplifications of the PIK3CA gene in thyroid tumors. *J Clin Endocrinol Metab*. 2005; 90 (9): 5509.

[21]   Wu G, Mambo E, Guo Z, Hu S, Huang X, Gollin SM, et al. Uncommon mutation, but common amplifications, of the PIK3CA gene in thyroid tumors. *J Clin Endocrinol Metab*. 2005; 90 (8): 4688-4693.

[22]   Ricarte-Filho JC, Ryder M, Chitale DA, Rivera M, Heguy A, Ladanyi M, et al. Mutational profile of advanced primary and metastatic radioactive iodine-refractory thyroid cancers reveals distinct pathogenetic roles for BRAF, PIK3CA, and AKT1. *Cancer Res*. 2009; 69 (11): 4885-4893.

[23]   Fagin JA. Challenging dogma in thyroid cancer molecular genetics--role of RET/PTC and BRAF in tumor initiation. *J Clin Endocrinol Metab*. 2004; 89 (9): 4264-4266.

[24]   Lemoine NR, Mayall ES, Wyllie FS, Williams ED, Goyns M, Stringer B, et al. High frequency of ras oncogene activation in all stages of human thyroid tumorigenesis. *Oncogene*. 1989; 4 (2): 159-164.

[25] Xing M. BRAF mutation in papillary thyroid cancer: pathogenic role, molecular bases, and clinical implications. *Endocr Rev.* 2007; 28 (7): 742-762.

[26] Rabes HM, Demidchik EP, Sidorow JD, Lengfelder E, Beimfohr C, Hoelzel D, et al. Pattern of radiation-induced RET and NTRK1 rearrangements in 191 post-chernobyl papillary thyroid carcinomas: biological, phenotypic, and clinical implications. *Clin Cancer Res.* 2000; 6 (3): 1093-1103.

[27] Rodriguez-Antona C, Pallares J, Montero-Conde C, Inglada-Perez L, Castelblanco E, Landa I, et al. Overexpression and activation of EGFR and VEGFR2 in medullary thyroid carcinomas is related to metastasis. *Endocr Relat Cancer.* 2010; 17 (1): 7-16.

[28] Martinez VD, Vucic EA, Becker-Santos DD, Gil L, Lam WL. Arsenic exposure and the induction of human cancers. *J Toxicol.* 2011; 2011 431287.

[29] Tokar EJ, Qu W, Waalkes MP. Arsenic, stem cells, and the developmental basis of adult cancer. *Toxicol Sci.* 2011; 120 Suppl 1 S192-203.

[30] Hippert MM, O'Toole PS, Thorburn A. Autophagy in cancer: good, bad, or both? *Cancer Res.* 2006; 66 (19): 9349-9351.

[31] Kimmelman AC. The dynamic nature of autophagy in cancer. *Genes & development.* 2011; 25 (19): 1999-2010.

[32] Huang YC, Hung WC, Chen WT, Yu HS, Chai CY. Sodium arsenite-induced DAPK promoter hypermethylation and autophagy via ERK1/2 phosphorylation in human uroepithelial cells. *Chem Biol Interact.* 2009; 181 (2): 254-262.

[33] Chai CY, Huang YC, Hung WC, Kang WY, Chen WT. Arsenic salts induced autophagic cell death and hypermethylation of DAPK promoter in SV-40 immortalized human uroepithelial cells. *Toxicol. Lett.* 2007; 173 (1): 48-56.

[34] Watcharasit P, Visitnonthachai D, Suntararuks S, Thiantanawat A, Satayavivad J. Low arsenite concentrations induce cell proliferation via activation of VEGF signaling in human neuroblastoma SH-SY5Y cells. *Environ Toxicol Pharmacol.* 2012; 33 (1): 53-59.

[35] Miller WH, Jr., Schipper HM, Lee JS, Singer J, Waxman S. Mechanisms of action of arsenic trioxide. *Cancer Res.* 2002; 62 (14): 3893-3903.

[36] Yang CH, Kuo ML, Chen JC, Chen YC. Arsenic trioxide sensitivity is associated with low level of glutathione in cancer cells. *Br J Cancer.* 1999; 81 (5): 796-799.

[37] Maeda H, Hori S, Nishitoh H, Ichijo H, Ogawa O, Kakehi Y, et al. Tumor growth inhibition by arsenic trioxide (As2O3) in the orthotopic metastasis model of androgen-independent prostate cancer. *Cancer Res.* 2001; 61 (14): 5432-5440.

[38] Chun YJ, Park IC, Park MJ, Woo SH, Hong SI, Chung HY, et al. Enhancement of radiation response in human cervical cancer cells in vitro and in vivo by arsenic trioxide (As2O3). *FEBS Lett.* 2002; 519 (1-3): 195-200.

[39] Vuky J, Yu R, Schwartz L, Motzer RJ. Phase II trial of arsenic trioxide in patients with metastatic renal cell carcinoma. *Invest New Drugs.* 2002; 20 (3): 327-330.

[40] Augustyns K, Bal G, Thonus G, Belyaev A, Zhang XM, Bollaert W, et al. The unique properties of dipeptidyl-peptidase IV (DPP IV / CD26) and the therapeutic potential of DPP IV inhibitors. *Curr Med Chem.* 1999; 6 (4): 311-327.

[41] Kindler HL, Aklilu M, Nattam S, Vokes EE. Arsenic trioxide in patients with adenocarcinoma of the pancreas refractory to gemcitabine: a phase II trial of the University of Chicago Phase II Consortium. *Am J Clin Oncol.* 2008; 31 (6): 553-556.

[42] Bael TE, Peterson BL, Gollob JA. Phase II trial of arsenic trioxide and ascorbic acid with temozolomide in patients with metastatic melanoma with or without central nervous system metastases. *Melanoma Res*. 2008; 18 (2): 147-151.

[43] Subbarayan PR, Lima M, Ardalan B. Arsenic trioxide/ascorbic acid therapy in patients with refractory metastatic colorectal carcinoma: a clinical experience. *Acta Oncol*. 2007; 46 (4): 557-561.

[44] Gallagher R, Ferrari A, Kaubisch A, Makower D, Stein C, Rajdev L, et al. Arsenic trioxide (ATO) in metastatic hormone-refractory prostate cancer (HRPC): Results of phase II trial T99–0077. *J Clin Oncol*. 2004; 22,14S 4638.

[45] Cohen KJ, Gibbs IC, Fisher PG, Hayashi RJ, Macy ME, Gore L. A phase I trial of arsenic trioxide chemoradiotherapy for infiltrating astrocytomas of childhood. *Neuro Oncol*. 2013; 15 (6): 783-787.

[46] Grimm SA, Marymont M, Chandler JP, Muro K, Newman SB, Levy RM, et al. Phase I study of arsenic trioxide and temozolomide in combination with radiation therapy in patients with malignant gliomas. *J Neurooncol*. 2012; 110 (2): 237-243.

[47] Tarhini AA, Kirkwood JM, Tawbi H, Gooding WE, Islam MF, Agarwala SS. Safety and efficacy of arsenic trioxide for patients with advanced metastatic melanoma. *Cancer*. 2008; 112 (5): 1131-1138.

[48] Huilgol NG. A phase I study to study arsenic trioxide with radiation and hyperthermia in advanced head and neck cancer. *Int J Hyperthermia*. 2006; 22 (5): 391-397.

[49] Ardalan B, Subbarayan PR, Ramos Y, Gonzalez M, Fernandez A, Mezentsev D, et al. A phase I study of 5-fluorouracil/leucovorin and arsenic trioxide for patients with refractory/relapsed colorectal carcinoma. *Clin Cancer Res*. 2010; 16 (11): 3019-3027.

[50] Podolsky L, Oh M, Subbarayan PR, Francheschi D, Livingstone A, Ardalan B. 5-Fluorouracil/Leucovorin and arsenic trioxide for patients with refractory/relapsed colorectal carcinoma: a clinical experience. *Acta Oncol*. 2011; 50 (4): 602-605.

[51] Qu FL, Hao XZ, Qin SK, Liu JW, Sui GJ, Chen Q, et al. [Multicenter phase II clinical trial of arsenic trioxide injection in the treatment of primary hepatocarcinoma]. *Chin J Oncol*. 2011; 33 (9): 697-701.

[52] Lin CC, Hsu C, Hsu CH, Hsu WL, Cheng AL, Yang CH. Arsenic trioxide in patients with hepatocellular carcinoma: a phase II trial. *Invest New Drugs*. 2007; 25 (1): 77-84.

[53] Bajorin DF, Halabi S, Small E. Arsenic trioxide in recurrent urothelial cancer: a cancer and leukemia group B phase II trial (CALGB 99903). *Clin Genitourin Cancer*. 2009; 7 (3): E66-70.

[54] Beer TM, Tangen CM, Nichols CR, Margolin KA, Dreicer R, Stephenson WT, et al. Southwest Oncology Group phase II study of arsenic trioxide in patients with refractory germ cell malignancies. *Cancer*. 2006; 106 (12): 2624-2629.

[55] Lai YL, Chang HH, Huang MJ, Chang KH, Su WH, Chen HW, et al. Combined effect of topical arsenic trioxide and radiation therapy on skin-infiltrating lesions of breast cancer-a pilot study. *Anticancer Drugs*. 2003; 14 (10): 825-828.

[56] Kim KB, Bedikian AY, Camacho LH, Papadopoulos NE, McCullough C. A phase II trial of arsenic trioxide in patients with metastatic melanoma. *Cancer*. 2005; 104 (8): 1687-1692.

[57] Ahn RW, Chen F, Chen H, Stern ST, Clogston JD, Patri AK, et al. A novel nanoparticulate formulation of arsenic trioxide with enhanced therapeutic efficacy in a murine model of breast cancer. *Clin Cancer Res*. 2010; 16 (14): 3607-3617.

[58] Yu H, Zhu GY, Xu RZ, Niu HZ, Lu Q, Li GZ, et al. Arterial embolization hyperthermia using As2O3 nanoparticles in VX2 carcinoma-induced liver tumors. *PloS one*. 2011; 6 (3): e17926.

[59] Printz C. Arsenic nanoparticle holds promise in blocking aggressive breast cancer. *Cancer*. 2010; 116 (24): 5567.

[60] Zhao S, Zhang X, Zhang J, Zou H, Liu Y, Dong X, et al. Intravenous administration of arsenic trioxide encapsulated in liposomes inhibits the growth of C6 gliomas in rat brains. *J Chemother*. 2008; 20 (2): 253-262.

[61] Li D, Du C, Lin Y, Wu M. Inhibition of growth of human nasopharyngeal cancer xenografts in SCID mice by arsenic trioxide. *Tumori*. 2002; 88 (6): 522-526.

[62] Yeh KY, Chang JW, Li YY, Wang CH, Wang HM. Tumor growth inhibition of metastatic nasopharyngeal carcinoma cell lines by low dose of arsenic trioxide via alteration of cell cycle progression and induction of apoptosis. *Head Neck*. 2011; 33 (5): 734-742.

[63] Pettersson HM, Pietras A, Munksgaard Persson M, Karlsson J, Johansson L, Shoshan MC, et al. Arsenic trioxide is highly cytotoxic to small cell lung carcinoma cells. *Mol Cancer Ther*. 2009; 8 (1): 160-170.

[64] Zhang J, Wang B. Arsenic trioxide (As(2)O(3)) inhibits peritoneal invasion of ovarian carcinoma cells in vitro and in vivo. *Gynecol Oncol*. 2006; 103 (1): 199-206.

[65] Wu DD, Xiao YF, Geng Y, Hou J. Antitumor effect and mechanisms of arsenic trioxide on subcutaneously implanted human gastric cancer in nude mice. *Cancer Genet Cytogenet*. 2010; 198 (2): 90-96.

[66] Zhao XS, Song PL, Sun B, Jiang HC, Liu TF. Arsenic trioxide inhibits metastatic potential of mouse hepatoma H22 cells in vitro and in vivo. *Hepatobil Pancreat Dis Int*. 2009; 8 (5): 510-517.

[67] Smith MA, Kang MH, Reynolds CP, Kurmasheva RT, Alexander D, Billups CA, et al. Evaluation of arsenic trioxide by the pediatric preclinical testing program with a focus on Ewing sarcoma. *Pediatr Blood Cancer*. 2012.

[68] Park WH, Kim SH. Arsenic trioxide induces human pulmonary fibroblast cell death via the regulation of Bcl-2 family and caspase-8. *Mol Biol Rep*. 2012; 39 (4): 4311-4318.

[69] Fröhlich E, Czarnocka B, Brossart P, Wahl R. Antitumor Effects of Arsenic Trioxide in Transformed Human Thyroid Cells. *Thyroid*. 2008; 18 (11): 1183-1193.

[70] Chen H, Ahn R, Van den Bossche J, Thompson DH, O'Halloran TV. Folate-mediated intracellular drug delivery increases the anticancer efficacy of nanoparticulate formulation of arsenic trioxide. *Mol Cancer Ther*. 2009; 8 (7): 1955-1963.

[71] Dilda PJ, Don AS, Tanabe KM, Higgins VJ, Allen JD, Dawes IW, et al. Mechanism of selectivity of an angiogenesis inhibitor from screening a genome-wide set of Saccharomyces cerevisiae deletion strains. *J Natl Cancer Inst*. 2005; 97 (20): 1539-1547.

[72] Eguchi R, Fujimori Y, Takeda H, Tabata C, Ohta T, Kuribayashi K, et al. Arsenic trioxide induces apoptosis through JNK and ERK in human mesothelioma cells. *J Cell Physiol*. 2011; 226 (3): 762-768.

[73] Kang YH, Lee SJ. The role of p38 MAPK and JNK in Arsenic trioxide-induced mitochondrial cell death in human cervical cancer cells. *J Cell Physiol*. 2008; 217 (1): 23-33.

[74]   Walker AM, Stevens JJ, Ndebele K, Tchounwou PB. Arsenic trioxide modulates DNA synthesis and apoptosis in lung carcinoma cells. *Int J Environ Res Public Health*. 2010; 7 (5): 1996-2007.

[75]   Chen H, Bai J, Ye J, Liu Z, Chen R, Mao W, et al. JWA as a functional molecule to regulate cancer cells migration via MAPK cascades and F-actin cytoskeleton. *Cell Signal*. 2007; 19 (6): 1315-1327.

[76]   Kim JH, Yu YS, Kim DH, Kim CJ, Kim KW. Antitumor activity of arsenic trioxide on retinoblastoma: cell differentiation and apoptosis depending on arsenic trioxide concentration. *Invest Ophthalmol Vis Sci*. 2009; 50 (4): 1819-1823.

[77]   Tingting R, Wei G, Changliang P, Xinchang L, Yi Y. Arsenic trioxide inhibits osteosarcoma cell invasiveness via MAPK signaling pathway. *Cancer Biol Ther*. 2010; 10 (3): 251-257.

[78]   Ray A, Roy S, Agarwal S, Bhattacharya S. As2O3 toxicity in rat hepatocytes: manifestation of caspase-mediated apoptosis. *Toxicol Ind Health*. 2008; 24 (10): 643-653.

[79]   Zanotto-Filho A, Braganhol E, Schroder R, de Souza LH, Dalmolin RJ, Pasquali MA, et al. NFkappaB inhibitors induce cell death in glioblastomas. *Biochem Pharmacol*. 2011; 81 (3): 412-424.

[80]   Zhang X, Su Y, Zhang M, Sun Z. Opposite effects of arsenic trioxide on the Nrf2 pathway in oral squamous cell carcinoma in vitro and in vivo. *Cancer Lett*. 2012; 318 (1): 93-98.

[81]   Wang XS, Wang GY, Xu HT, Wang K, Liu M, Fu SB, et al. [The effect of As2O3 on induction of apoptosis and inhibition of telomerase activity in colon cancer LS-174T cells]. *Chin J Oncol*. 2007; 29 (6): 415-418.

[82]   Zhou C, Boggess JF, Bae-Jump V, Gehrig PA. Induction of apoptosis and inhibition of telomerase activity by arsenic trioxide (As2O3) in endometrial carcinoma cells. *Gynecol Oncol*. 2007; 105 (1): 218-222.

[83]   Li Q, Bartlett DL, Gorry MC, O'Malley ME, Guo ZS. Three epigenetic drugs up-regulate homeobox gene Rhox5 in cancer cells through overlapping and distinct molecular mechanisms. *Mol Pharmacol*. 2009; 76 (5): 1072-1081.

[84]   Chen MJ, Yang PY, Ye YZ, Hu DN, Chen MF. Arsenic trioxide induces apoptosis in uveal melanoma cells through the mitochondrial pathway. *American journal of Chinese medicine*. 2010; 38 (6): 1131-1142.

[85]   Han YH, Kim SH, Kim SZ, Park WH. Apoptosis in arsenic trioxide-treated Calu-6 lung cells is correlated with the depletion of GSH levels rather than the changes of ROS levels. *J Cell Biochem*. 2008; 104 (3): 862-878.

[86]   Jutooru I, Chadalapaka G, Sreevalsan S, Lei P, Barhoumi R, Burghardt R, et al. Arsenic trioxide downregulates specificity protein (Sp) transcription factors and inhibits bladder cancer cell and tumor growth. *Exp Cell Res*. 2010; 316 (13): 2174-2188.

[87]   Paul MK, Kumar R, Mukhopadhyay AK. Dithiothreitol abrogates the effect of arsenic trioxide on normal rat liver mitochondria and human hepatocellular carcinoma cells. *Toxicol Appl Pharmacol*. 2008; 226 (2): 140-152.

[88]   Cheng B, Yang X, An L, Gao B, Liu X. Arsenic trioxide-induced apoptosis of Hep-2 cell line through modulating intracellular glutathione (GSH) level. *Auris, nasus, larynx*. 2010; 37 (1): 89-94.

[89] Raffoul F, Campla C, Nanjundan M. SnoN/SkiL, a TGFbeta signaling mediator: a participant in autophagy induced by arsenic trioxide. *Autophagy*. 2010; 6 (7): 955-957.

[90] Li Y, Tang LS, Shen HW. [Arsenic trioxide induced apoptosis in retinoblastoma cells in vitro and its possible mechanism]. *J Cent South Univ*. 2008; 33 (6): 476-480.

[91] Zhong F, Zhang S, Shao C, Yang J, Wu X. Arsenic trioxide inhibits cholangiocarcinoma cell growth and induces apoptosis. *Pathol Oncol Res*. 2010; 16 (3): 413-420.

[92] Cheng B, Yang X, Han Z, An L, Liu S. Arsenic trioxide induced the apoptosis of laryngeal cancer via down-regulation of survivin mRNA. *Auris, nasus, larynx*. 2008; 35 (1): 95-101.

[93] Yoo DR, Chong SA, Nam MJ. Proteome profiling of arsenic trioxide-treated human hepatic cancer cells. *Cancer genomics proteomics*. 2009; 6 (5): 269-274.

[94] Hou P, Liu D, Shan Y, Hu S, Studeman K, Condouris S, et al. Genetic alterations and their relationship in the phosphatidylinositol 3-kinase/Akt pathway in thyroid cancer. *Clin Cancer Res*. 2007; 13 (4): 1161-1170.

[95] Yu J, Qian H, Li Y, Wang Y, Zhang X, Liang X, et al. Therapeutic effect of arsenic trioxide (As2O3) on cervical cancer in vitro and in vivo through apoptosis induction. *Cancer Biol Ther*. 2007; 6 (4): 580-586.

[96] Yang GF, Li XH, Zhao Z, Wang WB. Arsenic trioxide up-regulates Fas expression in human osteosarcoma cells. *Chin Med J*. 2010; 123 (13): 1768-1773.

[97] Wen X, Li D, Zhang Y, Liu S, Ghali L, Iles RK. Arsenic trioxide induces cervical cancer apoptosis, but specifically targets human papillomavirus-infected cell populations. *Anti-cancer drugs*. 2012; 23 (3): 280-287.

[98] Wang X, Gao P, Long M, Lin F, Wei JX, Ren JH, et al. Essential role of cell cycle regulatory genes p21 and p27 expression in inhibition of breast cancer cells by arsenic trioxide. *Med Oncol*. 2011; 28 (4): 1225-1254.

[99] Xiao YF, Wu DD, Liu SX, Chen X, Ren LF. Effect of arsenic trioxide on vascular endothelial cell proliferation and expression of vascular endothelial growth factor receptors Flt-1 and KDR in gastric cancer in nude mice. *World J Gastroenterol*. 2007; 13 (48): 6498-6505.

[100] Xiao YF, Chen X, Liu SX, Wu DD, Ren LF. [Effect of arsenic trioxide on vascular endothelial growth factor-C and its receptor (VEGFR-3) in nude mice with gastric cancer]. *J Exp Hematol*. 2008; 16 (6): 1303-1307.

[101] Ai Z, Pan H, Suo T, Lv C, Wang Y, Tong S, et al. Arsenic oxide targets stem cell marker CD133/prominin-1 in gallbladder carcinoma. *Cancer Lett*. 2011; 310 (2): 181-187.

[102] Zhang S, Guo W, Ren TT, Lu XC, Tang GQ, Zhao FL. Arsenic trioxide inhibits Ewing's sarcoma cell invasiveness by targeting p38(MAPK) and c-Jun N-terminal kinase. *Anti-cancer drugs*. 2012; 23 (1): 108-118.

[103] Zhao H, Guo W, Peng C, Ji T, Lu X. Arsenic trioxide inhibits the growth of adriamycin resistant osteosarcoma cells through inducing apoptosis. *Mol Biol Rep*. 2010; 37 (5): 2509-2515.

[104] Du J, Zhou N, Liu H, Jiang F, Wang Y, Hu C, et al. Arsenic Induces Functional Re-Expression of Estrogen Receptor alpha by Demethylation of DNA in Estrogen Receptor-Negative Human Breast Cancer. *PloS one*. 2012; 7 (4): e35957.

[105] Zhang W, Wang L, Fan Q, Wu X, Wang F, Wang R, et al. Arsenic trioxide re-sensitizes ERalpha-negative breast cancer cells to endocrine therapy by restoring ERalpha expression in vitro and in vivo. *Oncol Rep.* 2011; 26 (3): 621-628.

[106] Chen GC, Guan LS, Hu WL, Wang ZY. Functional repression of estrogen receptor a by arsenic trioxide in human breast cancer cells. *Anticancer Res.* 2002; 22 (2A): 633-638.

[107] Davey JC, Bodwell JE, Gosse JA, Hamilton JW. Arsenic as an endocrine disruptor: effects of arsenic on estrogen receptor-mediated gene expression in vivo and in cell culture. *Toxicol Sci.* 2007; 98 (1): 75-86.

[108] Bae-Jump VL, Zhou C, Boggess JF, Gehrig PA. Arsenic trioxide (As2O3) inhibits expression of estrogen receptor-alpha through regulation of the mitogen-activated protein kinase (MAPK) pathway in endometrial cancer cells. *Reprod Sci.* 2008; 15 (10): 1011-1017.

[109] Sun H, Zhang S. Arsenic trioxide regulates the apoptosis of glioma cell and glioma stem cell via down-regulation of stem cell marker Sox2. *Biochem Biophys Res Commun.* 2011; 410 (3): 692-697.

[110] Zhang KZ, Zhang QB, Zhang QB, Sun HC, Ao JY, Chai ZT, et al. Arsenic trioxide induces differentiation of CD133+ hepatocellular carcinoma cells and prolongs posthepatectomy survival by targeting GLI1 expression in a mouse model. *J Hematol Oncol.* 2014; 7 28.

[111] Han JB, Sang F, Chang JJ, Hua YQ, Shi WD, Tang LH, et al. Arsenic trioxide inhibits viability of pancreatic cancer stem cells in culture and in a xenograft model via binding to SHH-Gli. *Onco Targets Ther.* 2013; 6 1129-1138.

[112] Carmignani M, Volpe AR, Aldea M, Soritau O, Irimie A, Florian IS, et al. Glioblastoma stem cells: a new target for metformin and arsenic trioxide. *J Biol Regul Homeost Agents.* 2014; 28 (1): 1-15.

[113] Ong PS, Chan SY, Ho PC. Differential augmentative effects of buthionine sulfoximine and ascorbic acid in As2O3-induced ovarian cancer cell death: oxidative stress-independent and -dependent cytotoxic potentiation. *Int J Oncol.* 2011; 38 (6): 1731-1739.

[114] Huang CY, Chen JY, Wu JE, Pu YS, Liu GY, Pan MH, et al. Ling-Zhi polysaccharides potentiate cytotoxic effects of anticancer drugs against drug-resistant urothelial carcinoma cells. *J Agr Food Chem.* 2010; 58 (15): 8798-8805.

[115] Li H, Zhu X, Zhang Y, Xiang J, Chen H. Arsenic trioxide exerts synergistic effects with cisplatin on non-small cell lung cancer cells via apoptosis induction. *J Exp Clin Cancer Res.* 2009; 28 110.

[116] Gunes DA, Florea AM, Splettstoesser F, Busselberg D. Co-application of arsenic trioxide (As2O3) and cisplatin (CDDP) on human SY-5Y neuroblastoma cells has differential effects on the intracellular calcium concentration ([Ca2+]i) and cytotoxicity. *Neurotoxicology.* 2009; 30 (2): 194-202.

[117] Zhang N, Wu ZM, McGowan E, Shi J, Hong ZB, Ding CW, et al. Arsenic trioxide and cisplatin synergism increase cytotoxicity in human ovarian cancer cells: therapeutic potential for ovarian cancer. *Cancer Sci.* 2009; 100 (12): 2459-2464.

[118] Lee PC, Kakadiya R, Su TL, Lee TC. Combination of bifunctional alkylating agent and arsenic trioxide synergistically suppresses the growth of drug-resistant tumor cells. *Neoplasia.* 2010; 12 (5): 376-387.

[119] Chung WH, Sung BH, Kim SS, Rhim H, Kuh HJ. Synergistic interaction between tetra-arsenic oxide and paclitaxel in human cancer cells in vitro. *Int J Oncol.* 2009; 34 (6): 1669-1679.

[120] Tomuleasa C, Soritau O, Fischer-Fodor E, Pop T, Susman S, Mosteanu O, et al. Arsenic trioxide plus cisplatin/interferon alpha-2b/doxorubicin/capecitabine combination chemotherapy for unresectable hepatocellular carcinoma. *Hematol Oncol Stem Cell Ther.* 2011; 4 (2): 60-66.

[121] Tomuleasa C, Soritau O, Kacso G, Fischer-Fodor E, Cocis A, Ioani H, et al. Arsenic trioxide sensitizes cancer stem cells to chemoradiotherapy. A new approach in the treatment of inoperable glioblastoma multiforme. *J BUON.* 2010; 15 (4): 758-762.

[122] Subbarayan PR, Lee K, Ardalan B. Arsenic trioxide suppresses thymidylate synthase in 5-FU-resistant colorectal cancer cell line HT29 In Vitro re-sensitizing cells to 5-FU. *Anticancer Res.* 2010; 30 (4): 1157-1162.

[123] Guilbert C, Annis MG, Dong Z, Siegel PM, Miller WH, Jr., Mann KK. Arsenic trioxide overcomes rapamycin-induced feedback activation of AKT and ERK signaling to enhance the anti-tumor effects in breast cancer. *PloS one.* 2013; 8 (12): e85995.

[124] Chien CW, Yao JH, Chang SY, Lee PC, Lee TC. Enhanced suppression of tumor growth by concomitant treatment of human lung cancer cells with suberoylanilide hydroxamic acid and arsenic trioxide. *Toxicol Appl Pharmacol.* 2011; 257 (1): 59-66.

[125] Wu J, Luo RC, Zhang H, Cui YZ. [Inhibitory effect of sorafenib combined with arsenic trioxide on hepatocellular carcinoma cells]. *J South Med Univ.* 2008; 28 (4): 639-641.

[126] Karsy M, Albert L, Murali R, Jhanwar-Uniyal M. The impact of arsenic trioxide and all-trans retinoic acid on p53 R273H-codon mutant glioblastoma. *Tumour Biol.* 2014; 35 (5): 4567-4580.

[127] Chen C, Zhang Y, Wang Y, Huang D, Xi Y, Qi Y. Synergic effect of 3'-azido-3'-deoxythymidine and arsenic trioxide in suppressing hepatoma cells. *Anti-cancer drugs.* 2011; 22 (5): 435-443.

[128] Shen P, Jiang T, Lu H, Han H, Luo R. Combination of Poly I:C and arsenic trioxide triggers apoptosis synergistically via activation of TLR3 and mitochondrial pathways in hepatocellular carcinoma cells. *Cell Biol Int.* 2011; 35 (8): 803-810.

[129] Wang W, Adachi M, Zhang R, Zhou J, Zhu D. A novel combination therapy with arsenic trioxide and parthenolide against pancreatic cancer cells. *Pancreas.* 2009; 38 (4): e114-123.

[130] Jin HO, Seo SK, Woo SH, Lee HC, Kim ES, Yoo DH, et al. A combination of sulindac and arsenic trioxide synergistically induces apoptosis in human lung cancer H1299 cells via c-Jun NH2-terminal kinase-dependent Bcl-xL phosphorylation. *Lung Cancer.* 2008; 61 (3): 317-327.

[131] Lee HR, Cheong HJ, Kim SJ, Lee NS, Park HS, Won JH. Sulindac enhances arsenic trioxide-mediated apoptosis by inhibition of NF-kappaB in HCT116 colon cancer cells. *Oncol Rep.* 2008; 20 (1): 41-47.

[132] Park JH, Kim EJ, Jang HY, Shim H, Lee KK, Jo HJ, et al. Combination treatment with arsenic trioxide and sulindac enhances apoptotic cell death in lung cancer cells via activation of oxidative stress and mitogen-activated protein kinases. *Oncol Rep.* 2008; 20 (2): 379-384.

[133] Sides MD, Sosulski ML, Luo F, Lin Z, Flemington EK, Lasky JA. Co-treatment with arsenic trioxide and ganciclovir reduces tumor volume in a murine xenograft model of nasopharyngeal carcinoma. *Virol J.* 2013; 10 152.

[134] Kim DW, Ahan SH, Kim TY. Enhancement of Arsenic Trioxide (As(2)O(3))- Mediated Apoptosis Using Berberine in Human Neuroblastoma SH-SY5Y Cells. *J Korean Neurosurg Soc.* 2007; 42 (5): 392-399.

[135] Lin TH, Kuo HC, Chou FP, Lu FJ. Berberine enhances inhibition of glioma tumor cell migration and invasiveness mediated by arsenic trioxide. *BMC Cancer.* 2008; 8 58.

[136] Chen G, Wang K, Yang BY, Tang B, Chen JX, Hua ZC. Synergistic antitumor activity of oridonin and arsenic trioxide on hepatocellular carcinoma cells. *Int J Oncol.* 2012; 40 (1): 139-147.

[137] Dizaji MZ, Malehmir M, Ghavamzadeh A, Alimoghaddam K, Ghaffari SH. Synergistic effects of arsenic trioxide and silibinin on apoptosis and invasion in human glioblastoma U87MG cell line. *Neurochem Res.* 2012; 37 (2): 370-380.

[138] Ting HC, Yen CC, Chen WK, Chang WH, Chou MC, Lu FJ. Humic acid enhances the cytotoxic effects of arsenic trioxide on human cervical cancer cells. *Environ Toxicol Pharmacol.* 2010; 29 (2): 117-125.

[139] Lee WJ, Lu FJ, Wang SF, Chen YR, Tseng TH. In vitro enhancement effect of humic acid on the progression of lung cancer cells. *Chem Biol Interact.* 2009; 181 (3): 463-471.

[140] Li W, Wang M, Wang L, Ji S, Zhang J, Zhang C. Icariin synergizes with arsenic trioxide to suppress human hepatocellular carcinoma. *Cell Biochem Biophys.* 2014; 68 (2): 427-436.

[141] Chiu HW, Lin W, Ho SY, Wang YJ. Synergistic effects of arsenic trioxide and radiation in osteosarcoma cells through the induction of both autophagy and apoptosis. *Radiat Res.* 2011; 175 (5): 547-560.

[142] Chiu HW, Chen YA, Ho SY, Wang YJ. Arsenic trioxide enhances the radiation sensitivity of androgen-dependent and -independent human prostate cancer cells. *PloS one.* 2012; 7 (2): e31579.

[143] Chiu HW, Ho SY, Guo HR, Wang YJ. Combination treatment with arsenic trioxide and irradiation enhances autophagic effects in U118-MG cells through increased mitotic arrest and regulation of PI3K/Akt and ERK1/2 signaling pathways. *Autophagy.* 2009; 5 (4): 472-483.

[144] Kumar P, Gao Q, Ning Y, Wang Z, Krebsbach PH, Polverini PJ. Arsenic trioxide enhances the therapeutic efficacy of radiation treatment of oral squamous carcinoma while protecting bone. *Mol Cancer Ther.* 2008; 7 (7): 2060-2069.

[145] Lew YS, Kolozsvary A, Brown SL, Kim JH. Synergistic interaction with arsenic trioxide and fractionated radiation in locally advanced murine tumor. *Cancer Res.* 2002; 62 (15): 4202-4205.

[146] Xie LX, Lin XH, Li DR, Chen JY, Hong CQ, Du CW. Synergistic therapeutic effect of arsenic trioxide and radiotherapy in BALB/C nude mice bearing nasopharyngeal carcinoma xenografts. *Exp Oncol.* 2007; 29 (1): 45-48.

[147] Diepart C, Karroum O, Magat J, Feron O, Verrax J, Calderon PB, et al. Arsenic trioxide treatment decreases the oxygen consumption rate of tumor cells and radiosensitizes solid tumors. *Cancer Res.* 2012; 72 (2): 482-490.

[148] Griffin RJ, Williams BW, Koonce NA, Bischof JC, Song CW, Asur R, et al. Vascular disrupting agent arsenic trioxide enhances thermoradiotherapy of solid tumors. *J Oncol.* 2012; 2012 934918.

[149] Wang L, Zhang J, An Y, Wang Z, Liu J, Li Y, et al. A study on the thermochemotherapy effect of nanosized As2O3/MZF thermosensitive magnetoliposomes on experimental hepatoma in vitro and in vivo. *Nanotechnology.* 2011; 22 (31): 315102.

[150] Wang ZY, Song J, Zhang DS. Nanosized As2O3/Fe2O3 complexes combined with magnetic fluid hyperthermia selectively target liver cancer cells. *World J Gastroenterol.* 2009; 15 (24): 2995-3002.

[151] Unnikrishnan D, Dutcher JP, Varshneya N, Lucariello R, Api M, Garl S, et al. Torsades de pointes in 3 patients with leukemia treated with arsenic trioxide. *Blood.* 2001; 97 (5): 1514-1516.

[152] Ling YH, Jiang JD, Holland JF, Perez-Soler R. Arsenic trioxide produces polymerization of microtubules and mitotic arrest before apoptosis in human tumor cell lines. *Mol Pharmacol.* 2002; 62 (3): 529-538.

[153] Han YH, Moon HJ, You BR, Kim SZ, Kim SH, Park WH. Effects of arsenic trioxide on cell death, reactive oxygen species and glutathione levels in different cell types. *Int J Mol Med.* 2010; 25 (1): 121-128.

[154] Stevens JJ, Graham B, Walker AM, Tchounwou PB, Rogers C. The effects of arsenic trioxide on DNA synthesis and genotoxicity in human colon cancer cells. *Int J Environ Res Public Health.* 2010; 7 (5): 2018-2032.

[155] Ouyang W, Li J, Ma Q, Huang C. Essential roles of PI-3K/Akt/IKKbeta/NFkappaB pathway in cyclin D1 induction by arsenite in JB6 Cl41 cells. *Carcinogenesis.* 2006; 27 (4): 864-873.

[156] Pochin EE. Prospects from the treatment of thyroid carcinoma with radioiodine. *Clin Radiol.* 1967; 18 (2): 113-125.

[157] Antonelli A, Fallahi P, Ferrari SM, Ruffilli I, Santini F, Minuto M, et al. New targeted therapies for thyroid cancer. *Current genomics.* 2011; 12 (8): 626-631.

[158] Sherman SI. Targeted therapies for thyroid tumors. *Mod Pathol.* 2011; 24 Suppl 2 S44-52.

[159] Brose MS, Nutting CM, Sherman SI, Shong YK, Smit JW, Reike G, et al. Rationale and design of decision: a double-blind, randomized, placebo-controlled phase III trial evaluating the efficacy and safety of sorafenib in patients with locally advanced or metastatic radioactive iodine (RAI)-refractory, differentiated thyroid cancer. *BMC Cancer.* 2011; 11 349.

[160] Brose M, Nutting C, Jarzab B, Elisei R, Siena S, Bastholt L, et al. Sorafenib in locally advanced or metastatic patients with radioactive iodine-refractory differentiated thyroid cancer: The phase III DECISION trial. *J Clin Oncol.* 2013 31 (suppl; abstr 4).

[161] Hayes DN, Lucas AS, Tanvetyanon T, Krzyzanowska MK, Chung CH, Murphy B, et al. Phase II efficacy and pharmacogenomic study of selumetinib (AZD6244; ARRY-142886) in iodine-131 refractory papillary thyroid carcinoma (IRPTC) with or without follicular elements. *Clin Cancer Res.* 2012; 18 (7): 2056-2065.

[162] Ho AL, Grewal RK, Leboeuf R, Sherman EJ, Pfister DG, Deandreis D, et al. Selumetinib-enhanced radioiodine uptake in advanced thyroid cancer. *New Engl J Med.* 2013; 368 (7): 623-632.

[163] Woyach JA, Kloos RT, Ringel MD, Arbogast D, Collamore M, Zwiebel JA, et al. Lack of therapeutic effect of the Histone Deacetylase Inhibitor Vorinostat in Patients with Metastatic Radioiodine-Refractory Thyroid Carcinoma. *J Clin Endocrinol Metab*. 2008; 94 (1): 164-170.

[164] Sherman E, Fury M, Tuttle R, Ghossein R, Stambuk H, Baum M, et al. Phase II study of depsipeptide (DEP) in radioiodine (RAI)-refractory metastatic nonmedullary thyroid carcinoma. *Proc Am Soc Clin Oncol*. 2009; 27 (15s): 6059.

[165] Zhang Y, Jia S, Liu Y, Li B, Wang Z, Lu H, et al. A clinical study of all-trans-retinoid-induced differentiation therapy of advanced thyroid cancer. *Nucl Med Commun*. 2007; 28 (4): 251-255.

[166] Kim WG, Kim EY, Kim TY, Ryu JS, Hong SJ, Kim WB, et al. Redifferentiation therapy with 13-cis retinoic acids in radioiodine-resistant thyroid cancer. *Endocr J*. 2009; 56 (1): 105-112.

[167] Handkiewicz-Junak D, Roskosz J, Hasse-Lazar K, Szpak-Ulczok S, Puch Z, Kukulska A, et al. 13-cis-retinoic acid re-differentiation therapy and recombinant human thyrotropin-aided radioiodine treatment of non-Functional metastatic thyroid cancer: a single-center, 53-patient phase 2 study. *Thyroid Res*. 2009; 2 (1): 8.

[168] Kebebew E, Lindsay S, Clark OH, Woeber KA, Hawkins R, Greenspan FS. Results of rosiglitazone therapy in patients with thyroglobulin-positive and radioiodine-negative advanced differentiated thyroid cancer. *Thyroid*. 2009; 19 (9): 953-956.

[169] Kebebew E, Peng M, Reiff E, Treseler P, Woeber KA, Clark OH, et al. A phase II trial of rosiglitazone in patients with thyroglobulin-positive and radioiodine-negative differentiated thyroid cancer. *Surgery*. 2006; 140 (6): 960-966.

[170] Tepmongkol S, Keelawat S, Honsawek S, Ruangvejvorachai P. Rosiglitazone effect on radioiodine uptake in thyroid carcinoma patients with high thyroglobulin but negative total body scan: a correlation with the expression of peroxisome proliferator-activated receptor-gamma. *Thyroid*. 2008; 18 (7): 697-704.

[171] Fröhlich E, Wahl R. The current role of targeted therapies to induce radioiodine uptake in thyroid cancer. *Cancer Treat Rev*. 2014; 40 (5): 665-674.

[172] Tuttle RM, Rondeau G, Lee NY. A risk-adapted approach to the use of radioactive iodine and external beam radiation in the treatment of well-differentiated thyroid cancer. *Cancer control*. 2011; 18 (2): 89-95.

[173] Brierley J, Sherman E. The role of external beam radiation and targeted therapy in thyroid cancer. *Semin Radiat Oncol*. 2012; 22 (3): 254-262.

[174] Marx K, Moka D, Schomacker K, Fischer T, Gabruk-Szostak B, Kobe C, et al. Cell death induced by 131 I in a differentiated thyroid carcinoma cell line in vitro: necrosis or apoptosis? *Nucl Med Commun*. 2006; 27 (4): 353-358.

[175] Baskar R, Lee KA, Yeo R, Yeoh KW. Cancer and radiation therapy: current advances and future directions. *Int J Med Sci*. 2012; 9 (3): 193-199.

[176] Nehs MA, Lin CI, Kozono DE, Whang EE, Cho NL, Zhu K, et al. Necroptosis is a novel mechanism of radiation-induced cell death in anaplastic thyroid and adrenocortical cancers. *Surgery*. 2011; 150 (6): 1032-1039.

In: Horizons in Cancer Research. Volume 55
Editor: Hiroto S. Watanabe

ISBN: 978-1-63463-228-7
© 2015 Nova Science Publishers, Inc.

Chapter 4

Xerostomia: Causes, Prevention and Management

Hong Wu, M.D., M.S.[1,2], Jennifer Yacub Martin, M.D.[1]
and Dian Wang, M.D., Ph.D.[3]

[1]Department of Physical Medicine and Rehabilitation,
Medical College of Wisconsin, US
[2]Department of Anesthesiology,
Medical College of Wisconsin, US
[3]Department of Radiation Oncology,
Medical College of Wisconsin, US

Abstract

Xerostomia, the subjective perception of dry mouth, is due to a variety of etiologies including polypharmacy, chemoradiation of head and neck cancers, systemic diseases and autoimmune disorders. It is associated with impaired swallowing, speech, taste, oral health, sleep and nutrition and thus can have a significant impact on a patient's quality of life. Given the significant effects of xerostomia, prevention and management of this symptom are of great importance in clinical practice. Prevention strategies are aimed at reducing the severity of xerostomia and are thus focused on reduction of radiation exposure, cytoprotectants, secretagogues and submandibular gland transfers. Treatment of xerostomia is challenging and unfortunately is not curative. Options for treatment include pharmacological agents, salivary substitutes, acupuncture, hyperbaric oxygen therapy, stimulants, oral care, and treatment of the underlying systemic or autoimmune disorder. Future investigations include gene transfer/therapy and stem cell replacement. The purpose of this chapter is to outline the causes, prevention and evidence based management of xerostomia to guide this undertreated clinical condition.

Introduction

Xerostomia is defined as dry mouth resulting from reduced or absent saliva flow [1, 2, 3]. The most common causes of xerostomia include medication side effects, chemoradiotherapy or radiation therapy for head and neck cancers, systemic diseases and autoimmune disorders and normal aging.

The clinical manifestations of xerostomia are vast and should be recognized by clinical professionals. Manifestations include a thin, pale oral cavity with cracked appearance that is susceptible to gingivitis and bleeding; a dry sticky mouth and nutritional deficiencies [1, 4]. Those with systemic causes of xerostomia may have enlarged parotids or submandibular glands. Patients may complain of a series of symptoms including dry throat, mouth, skin; sore throat/tongue; difficulty swallowing/speaking; altered taste (dysguesia); dry/burning eyes; dental decay; poor nutrition; inflammation and fissuring of the lips (chelitis); salivary gland infection (sialandenitis); halitosis; oral candidiasis and sleep disturbances due to frequent awakenings for water [1, 4, 5]. These symptoms may then lead to significant morbidity and diminished quality of life (QOL) [3]. Refer to Table 1 for a listing of common consequences of xerostomia.

Despite current treatment options, the prevention and treatment of xerostomia remains a clinical challenge. In this review we will list the common causes of xerostomia, discuss the prevention strategies and summarize the up-to-date and evidence based managements of xerostomia in order to improve the awareness of xerostomia and provide prevention and treatment options that can be implemented as indicated. Utilizing PubMed, a review of the published literature between the years 1990 and 2014 was conducted. The articles reviewed consist mostly of clinical trials, however a small number of case reports/series were included.

Table 1. Signs and Symptoms of Xerostomia

Signs	Symptoms
Dry throat, mouth, eye, skin	Dental decay/carries
Fissuring/inflammation of the lips, tongue	Gingivitis
Thick saliva	Altered taste (dysguesia)
Swelling of the salivary glands	Sleep disturbance
Candidiasis	Difficulty swallowing
	Difficulty speaking
	Poor nutrition

Pathogenesis and Etiology

Ninety percent of saliva is produced by the major salivary glands: parotid, submandibular and sublingual [1, 2]. The rest is produced by the minor salivary glands: lingual, labial, buccal, palatine, glossopalatine [1, 2]. In the unstimulated state the submandibular gland produces most of the saliva while in the stimulated state the parotid gland is responsible for the majority of the saliva produced [2, 6]. The secretory unit of the salivary gland consists of the acinar cells, myoepithelial cells, intercalacted ducts, striated ducts and excretory ducts [2].

There are two major salivary secretions: serous fluid and mucous fluid [1, 2]. Serous fluid is protein rich and contains bactericidal components whereas the mucous fluid is rich in glycoconjugates containing water and mucin which provide lubrication and prevent epithelial dehydration [1, 2]. It is the decline in mucin that results in xerostomia [1]. In healthy individuals, total salivary flow is up to 1.5 L per day [2]. Decreased salivary flow rate can be defined as unstimulated salivary flow rates < 0.1 ml/min or stimulated who saliva flow rate < 0.7 ml/min. The general consensus is to define xerostomia at a reduced salivary flow of at least 25 percent [2, 7] however, symptoms of xerostomia typically become evident when salivary flow decreases to around 50 percent of normal [1, 4].

The prevalence of xerostomia increases with age, however it should be noted that salivary gland hypo-functioning is not a normal part of aging [1]. Xerostomia is often associated with radiation therapy, autoimmune diseases, and medication use including chemo-agents, pain medications, anti-hypertensive medications and anti-psychotic medications. It is also related to systemic diseases such as diabetes mellitus, thyroid disorders, cystic fibrosis, connective tissue disorders, arthritis, perceived medical health, dependence in physical functioning, female gender and mouth breathing [1, 4].

There are two types of xerostomia: temporary and chronic. Temporary hyposalivation affects only resting salivary secretion and there is a maintained ability to react to gustatory and olfactory stimulation [1]. Temporary hyposalivation is most often attributed to drug induced xerostomia and should resolve with removal of the offending agent. Chronic hyposalivation affects resting and stimulated secretion rates, increases the rate of dental and oral mucosal disease and shows a decreased response to treatment [1]. Chronic hyposalivation is typically associated with systemic and autoimmune disorders. In this case the xerostomia is often irreversible; however symptoms may be controlled with treatment of the underlying disorder. The incidence of head and neck cancer (HNC) is about 5% of all the cancer in the world. Radiation therapy (RT) is an important treatment modality especially early-to-intermediate stage HNC and combined chemoradiotherapy is often given for locally advanced stage HNC [8]. Virtually all patients who undergo RT of HNC have some degree of xerostomia as a result of damage to the salivary glands [8, 9]. Xerostomia may also be caused or exacerbated by the concomitant or sequential use of chemotherapy agents and other drugs. The treatment induced xerostomia will often result in chronic hyposalivation as full recovery of the salivary gland tissue is unlikely. In addition to dry mouth, taste and swallowing can also be affected due to impaired modulation of saliva on taste and perception of swallowing. Saliva plays a significant role in taste acuity. A diminished salivary flow can markedly affect the modulating effects on the basic taste modalities: sour, sweet, salty, and bitter. Saliva strongly influences salt taste threshold levels and provides the ionic environment for taste cells through signal transduction. The type of taste stimuli can influence salivary flow rate and composition. Sour taste induces the highest flow rate and sodium concentrations, whereas salt gives rise to high protein and calcium concentrations. Chemoreceptors on the dorsal tongue anatomy are markedly affected by xerostomia with a diminished acuity, therefore decreasing the effect of taste and affecting the patient's quality of life [10, 11, 12].

Medications

Over four hundred medications have been implicated in contributing symptoms of dry mouth [13, 14]. The mechanism of medication induced salivary hypo-function is by inhibiting signaling pathways within salivary tissue and reducing fluid output in the gland [1, 14]. Since the salivary glands are strongly stimulated by cholinergic agents, anticholinergics are some of the most likely culprits of xerostomia [1, 4]. Other drug classes that are associated with xerostomia include pain medications, sedatives, antihistamines, antipsychotics, diuretics and antidepressants [1, 4].

Table 2. Medications associated with xerostomia [17]

Drug Class	Example(s)
Anorexiant (appetite suppressant)	Methamphetamine
Antiacne	Isotretinoin (oral preparation)
Antianxiety	Diazepam
Anticholinergic	Oxybutynin
Anticonvulsant	Gabapentin
Antidepressant	Amitriptyline (TCA*)
	Sertraline (SSRI*)
Antidiarrheal	Loperamide
Antiemetic	Ondansetron
Antihistamine	Loratadine
Antihypertensive	Enalapril (ACE*)
	Losartan (ARB*)
	Clonidine (Adrenergic Stimulant)
	Metoprolol (Beta Blocker)
	Amlodipine (CCB*)
	Hydrochlorothiazide (Thiazide)
	Furosemide (Loop Diuretic)
	Spironolactone (Potassium sparing)
Anti-inflammatory	Diclofenac (NSAID*)
	Fluticasone proprionate (Steorid)
Antiparkinsonism	Carbidopa/Levodopa
Antipsychotic	Clozapine
Antispasmodic	Baclofen
Bronchodilators	Albuterol
Decongestant	Pseudoephedrine
Narcotic analgesic	Morphine
Sedative	Temazepam
Chemoagents	5-fluorouracil, vinblastine,

*TCA= Tricyclic; SSRI= Selective Serotonin Reuptake Inhibitor; ACE= Angiotensin Converting Enzyme; ARB= Angiotensin Receptor Blocker; CCB= Calcium Channel Blocker; NSAID= Non-Steroidal Anti-Inflammatory.

Chemotherapy agents aim to destroy cancer cells, which reproduce very quickly, thus normal cells that multiply rapidly are equally susceptible to the effects of these drugs. Chemotherapeutic medications that are commonly used in the treatment of HNC and thus are associated with xerostomia include; 5-fluorouracil, vinblastine, cyclophosphamide, methotrexate, cisplatin and bleomycin [15, 16]. The dry mouth symptoms usually improve 2-

8 weeks following the chemotherapy. Patients who present with symptoms of xerostomia should also be asked about the use of non-prescription medications such as Ginkgo biloba, St. John's Wort, caffeine, garlic, capsicum and medications in the labiatate family as all of these classes have been associated with the incidence of xerostomia [4]. A summary of common medications that can induce xerostomia is listed in Table 2 [17].

Radiation

The most pronounced symptoms of xerostomia are in those patients who have had therapeutic irradiation for HNC [1]. Up to 100 percent of patients who have received radiation therapy for HNC have reported some degree of dry mouth [18]. The development of post radiation xerostomia is likely dependent on a variety of prognostic factors including radiation dose distribution, demographics, tumor-related and treatment-related factors [19].With regards to the location of radiation, most studies have focused on the effects of radiation to the parotid salivary glands as these glands produce nearly 60% of stimulated saliva [20]. The contribution of other salivary glands such as the submandibular gland is less well studied however more focus should be placed on these glands as radiation therapy to these locations have also been shown to correlate with patient reported xerostomia [20]. Lee et al showed that the radiation dose to the parotid glands was the only significant predictive factor of xerostomia [21]. Contrary to Lee's findings, Eisbruch et al demonstrated that the radiotherapy effect to the minor salivary glands is an independent predictor of xerostomia [22]. This finding thus suggests the need for a plan to spare not only the major salivary glands but also the noninvolved oral cavity including the minor salivary glands [22]. Eisbruch et al also demonstrated that the radiotherapy dose to the submandibular gland was a significant explanatory variable for the Xerostomia Questionnaire score difference (p=0.009), whereas the dose to the parotid gland was only marginally significant (p=0.05) [22].

Radiation induces cytotoxic injury to the salivary gland parenchyma and its vascular supply [1, 3]. This destruction inevitably results in impaired autonomic controls and hence dysfunctional acinar cells [3]. Damage to the plasma membrane of the acinar cells results in disruption of intracellular signal transduction, ultimately causing a change in salivary composition (ie- immunoglobulins, buffers, small organic molecules), consistency, volume and pH [2, 3, 11, 23]. Radiation also causes destruction of progenitor cells and stem cells which renders acinar cells non-functional over time [2, 3]. Further dysfunction occurs due to acinar cell degeneration, fibrosis, necrosis and atrophy [24]. The dysfunction of the acinar cells subsequently leads to salivary hypofunction which leads to acute and chronic xerostomia [1, 3]. Despite some regeneration, function remains indefinitely impaired due to damage to the blood vessels, ducts and nerves [3, 7]. Even with regeneration, flow rate and amylase production can continue to deteriorate [2, 3]. The degree of destruction depends on the dose of radiation administered [1]. Mean radiation doses between 20-40 Gray (Gy) to the parotid gland results in significant reduction in stimulated salivary flow rates with 50-60 % reduction occurring in the first week and reduction to nearly 20% by week seven of conventional radiation therapy [3, 24]. After a radiation dose of 40-42 Gy, salivary flow rate is often undetectable [2]. Destruction is often permanent, however unless the entire gland has undergone radiation, partial recovery is likely to occur within 6-12 months [1]. Adjunct chemotherapy using bleomycin, 5-fluorouracil, vinblastine, cyclophosphamide, methotrexate or cisplatin, induces acute toxicity and further increased salivary gland dysfunction (up to 70 percent) as compared to radiation alone [2, 15, 16].

Autoimmune Disorders

Sjogren's Syndrome (SS) is an autoimmune disorder that primarily affects the salivary and lacrimal glands causing clusters of infiltrating lymphocytes to replace the parenchyma of the glands [1, 13]. This change causes subsequent loss of secretory epithelial cells and thus changes the salivary flow rate and composition [1, 13]. SS typically affects middle aged and elderly white women but can occur in all ages and ethnic backgrounds [1]. In primary Sjogren's, xerostomia and keratoconjunctivitis sicca develop as isolated clinical entities whereas secondary Sjogren's occurs as a complication of a pre-existing connective tissue disease (ie- Rheumatoid Arthritis, Systemic Lupus Erythematous or Scleroderma) [1, 13]. The prevalence of primary Sjogren's Syndrome in the United States is noted to be 3 percent in those over age 50 and the prevalence of secondary Sjogren's is noted to be approximately 31.8% in those diagnosed with Mixed Connective Tissue Diseases (MCTD) [25, 26].

Another chronic inflammatory disease that leads to xerostomia is sarcoidosis. In this disease, non-caseating granulomas lead to the destruction of the salivary glands [1].

Other

Aside from the aforementioned causes of xerostomia other contributing factors to its development include cigarette use, dysgeusia, frequent snacking behavior, poorly controlled diabetes, chronic graft versus host disease, thyroid disorders, hepatitis C, Milkulicz's disease (a syndrome characterized by lymphocytic infiltration of glands in the head and neck), surgical removal of salivary glands, dehydration, psychogenic conditions (fear, anxiety, depression), mouth breathing, nasal obstruction, damage to head and neck causing damage to the nerves that innervate the salivary glands, candidiasis [1, 13]. Table 3 provides a summary of common causes of xerostomia.

Table 3. Etiology of xerostomia and associated conditions/diseases

Etiology	Associated Conditions/Diseases
Medications (seeTable II)	Diabetes
Radiation	Thyroid disorders
Continuous positive airway pressure (CPAP) device	Sleep apnea
Autoimmune disorders	Osteoarthritis
Sjogren syndrome	Cystic Fibrosis
Systemic Lupus Erythematous	Connective Tissue Disorders
Rheumatoid Arthritis	Psychogenic conditions (anxiety, depression)
Scleroderma	Hepatitis C
Sarcoidosis	Chronic graft versus host disease

Prevention

Reduce Radiation Exposure

Radiation delivery techniques that have been shown to improve radiation- induced xerostomia are intensity-modulated radiotherapy (IMRT) and 3-dimensional conformal radiotherapy both which aim to spare the adjacent normal tissues including salivary glands from high dose irradiation [3]. The parotid gland produces approximately 60 percent of salivary output in the stimulated state thus most studies have attempted to reduce the radiation dose to those glands [2]. Standard radiation therapy techniques may place the entire or uninvolved salivary glands at risk of exposure to radiation. In a phase I and II trial conducted at the University of Michigan, IMRT has been shown to reduce the radiation dose to the contralateral parotid gland to 32 percent compared with 93 percent in standard plans [2]. Spared parotid glands that received a mean dose of 19.9 Gy recovered 63 percent of their pretreatment stimulated flow rate at 1 year versus only 3 percent recovery for parotid glands that received 57.5 Gy [2]. Mean dose threshold for stimulated saliva flow rate is 26 Gy and 24 Gy in unstimulated saliva flow rates [2]. Studies have shown that glands receiving a mean dose below or equal to the threshold showed a substantial preservation of saliva flow after radiotherapy [2]. Glands that received doses above the mean threshold produced little saliva and had no recovery over time [2]. IMRT has been shown to significantly lessen the symptoms of xerostomia at rest and with meals and has improved xerostomia related QOL scores [24].

In a randomized control trial conducted by Pow et al, whole salivary flow rates and parotid salivary flow rates were significantly ($p<0.05$) higher in the IMRT group versus the conventional radiotherapy group (Pow et al). However, even with the use of IMRT the development of xerostomia remains high as IMRT only partly spares the parotid glands and minor salivary glands in certain HNC patients [22, 27, 28, 29, 30, 31]. Further potential disadvantages of IMRT include increased homogeneity of the dose distribution, increased total body dose, increased planning time, increased cost, the increased difficulty in interpretation of treatment verification films, the potentially increased risk of a marginal miss [28, 32] and the low availability (< 10 percent of the global population) [7].

Cytoprotectants

Amifostine (WR-1065) is the most widely used cytoprotectant [2]. It is an intracellular scavenger of free radicals that serves to protect subcellular structures such as membranes and DNA from damage [2, 24, 33]. In a phase III randomized control study conducted by Brizel et al; amifostine was administered to patients requiring definitive or postoperative radiation [34]. In this study amifostine was shown to reduce acute and chronic xerostomia without compromising anti-tumor efficacy [34]. Further phase III randomized trials demonstrated that both subcutaneous and intravenous administration of amifostine had equal efficacy in regards to cytotoxicity protection [35]. Regardless of its apparent benefits there has been some hesitation towards the widespread use of amifostine. There are studies which bring into question the potential tumor protective effect and toxicity of the drug as there may not be selective uptake of amifostine into normal tissue [2]. Aside from the question of its tumor protective effect amifostine has been noted to have side effects of hypotension, nausea, vomiting, allergic reactions and toxic epidermonecrolysis (Stevens Johnson Syndrome) [2, 7]. The American Society of Clinical Oncology has summarized the current evidence and has recommended the use of amifostine for the prevention of xerostomia during radiotherapy, but not chemoradiotherapy for HNC (Level II evidence, grade C recommendation) [2, 7]. Despite this recommendation amifostine is not always a treatment of choice due to cost; logistical problems given the need for subcutaneous or parenteral administration prior to each radiotherapy session and its lack of universal availability [7, 28, 34].

Secretogogues

These are parasympathomimetic, muscarinic agonists which induce a transient increase in salivary output and have been noted to have a statistically significant improvement on complaints of oral dryness [4]. Pilocarpine and Cevimeline are two pharmacological agents that have been studied in the management of xerostomia. Pilocarpine is approved by the FDA for the treatment of patients with head and neck radiation associated xerostomia, however there is only Level II evidence, grade C recommendation for its routine use in the prevention of xerostomia [4, 7]. Additionally, the benefits of pilocarpine may only be short term and there may be some intolerable side effects that accompany its use. Cevimeline has been studied in the use of SS associated xerostomia, but it is still investigational. See the section on 'Treatment' for further information regarding these two medications.

Submandibular Gland Transfer

The submandibular gland produces nearly 65 percent of unstimulated saliva [6] thus efforts aimed at the preservation of these glands may have a result in an improvement in xerostomia symptoms. Jha and Seiklay first reported good results on the prevention of radiation induced xerostomia by submandibular gland transfer in 2000 [36]. They described a method of transferring the submandibular gland to the submental space, an area that can be shielded from radiation and that does not have detrimental effects on cure rates in tumors distant from the submental triangle [36, 37, 38]. In this technique the submandibular gland receives only 5 percent of the total radiation dose and thus the damage to the gland is significantly reduced [39]. This technique was utilized in a prospective clinical randomized control study conducted by Zhang et al who found improvement in xerostomia symptoms-speech, chewing, swallowing, changes in eating habits, nighttime xerostomia, need to wake up to drink frequently and disturbed sleep quality- up to 60 months after treatment was completed [40]. The American Society of Clinical Oncology suggests that submandibular gland transfer may be of clinical significance (Level IV evidence, grade B recommendation) [7].

Other approaches to potentially reducing the risk of RT associated xerostomia include laser phototherapy to mucositis, intraglandular botulinum prior to RT (animal studies), daily dosing of alpha-tocopherol (vitamin E) supplementation and the plant alkaloid cepharanthin [24]. When administered prior to radiotherapy, intraglandular administration of botulinum toxin may lead to glandular involution with reduction of acinar granules for the time of irradiation and thus significantly reduce the radiation sensitivity [41]. Further studies are needed to examine the efficacy of botulinum toxin in the prevention of radiation induced xerostomia.

Preventative measures that should be initiated to minimize the effects and / or progression of xerostomia include: seeing a dental hygienist at least three times per year; brushing with fluoride toothpaste after each meal; low sugar intake and avoiding excess consumption of acidic beverages [4]. Dry, spicy and acidic foods should also be avoided as they can contribute mucosal irritation [42, 43, 44].

Treatment

Unfortunately exact course of xerostomia is unknown and the symptoms will rarely resolve completely [28]. Treatment options for xerostomia include muscarinic acetylcholine agonists (pilocarpine and cevilmeline); salivary substitutes; mechanical, gustatory and electrical salivary stimulants; acupuncture and hyperbaric oxygen therapy (HBOT) [3]. Despite the variety of options available there are no set guidelines for the treatment of xerostomia [3].

Pharmacological Treatments

Pilocarpine is a non-selective muscarinic receptor agonist and is the only treatment option approved by the US Food and Drug Administration for the treatment of radiation-induced salivary hypofunction [3, 7]. The likely mechanism of action is by causing the depletion of secretory granules in serous cells and reducing the extent of radiation-induced gland damage [7]. In a multicenter randomized, double-blind, placebo-controlled study conducted by LeVeque et al, pilocarpine was noted to significantly improve unstimulated parotid salivary rates after 12 weeks of treatment ($p<0.001$) [45]. These results were corroborated by the results of two prospective randomized control trials which reported a significant improvement in whole saliva and unstimulated parotid saliva production at 12 weeks ($p=0.003$ and $p<0.001$ respectively) [46]. In a meta-analysis compiled by Lovelace et al pilocarpine, particularly the pilocarpine lozenge demonstrated the best results when measuring increased unstimulated salivary flow rates [3]. In patients with xerostomia studies have demonstrated increased salivary flow rates within 15 minutes after administration of pilocarpine and peak flow rates have been shown to be maintained for at least 1 hour [13]. It has also been demonstrated that unstimulated whole salivary flow rates significantly increase over 3 to 6 months [47]. Despite this increase in salivary flow rates the patient's perception of dry mouth remains unchanged as assessed by a patient reported linear analog scale (LASA) [47, 48]. Despite obvious benefit pilocarpine is often discontinued due to its undesirable side effects which include sweating, chills, nausea, dizziness, rhinitis and asthenia [13]. It must also be noted that tolerance often develops while using pilocarpine and thus its efficacy will plateau. Additionally, Pilocarpine is contraindicated in patients with a history of bronchospasm, severe COPD, congestive heart disease, uncontrolled asthma, acute iritis and angle closure glaucoma [2, 3].

Cevimeline is a muscarinic acetylcholine receptor agonist. It has a high affinity for muscarinic M3 receptors that are found in the salivary glands [3]. Compared to pilocarpine it has been noted to have a longer half- life and duration of action and has fewer severe respiratory and cardiac adverse effects [2, 3]. In a randomized, placebo controlled trial conducted by Petrone et al, Cevimeline, administered at 30-45 mg three times daily for 52 weeks, was shown to significantly increase unstimulated saliva however it did not change the amount of stimulated saliva measured [49, 50]. Cevimeline has been approved in the United States to treat Sjogren's associated xerostomia; however it is not yet approved for radiation induced xerostomia [3].

Bethanechol is a cholinergic choline carbamate with mostly M3 muscarinic activity and thus similar to pilocarpine. It has been noted to have muscarinic side effects [3]. There are few studies on the efficacy of bethanechol on radiation induced hyposalivation, however those that have been conducted suggest it may provide some minimal improvement in salivary flow and subjective xerostomia [3, 7].

Anethole Trithione is another drug that has the potential to treat xerostomia in SS. It is a bile secretion-stimulating drug that stimulates the parasympathetic nervous systems thereby increasing the secretion of acetylcholine and subsequently stimulates salivary secretion from acinar cells [5]. It is often used in the treatment of chronic xerostomia at dose of 25 mg three times per day [5, 13]. Side effects include abdominal discomfort and flatulence [5]. There are differing reports of the effects of the medication however there are some reports that note increased salivary flow rates in drug induced xerostomia [5]. Synergistic effects between the concurrent use of pilocarpine and anethole trithione have been reported however further studies are needed to delineate the true safety and efficacy of anethole trithione [5, 13].

Other drugs that can stimulate the salivary glands include carbamylcholine, neostigmine, pyridostigmine and yohimbine (an alpha 2 adrenergic antagonist which can be helpful in drug induced oral dryness). Unfortunately there is a lack of research supporting the efficacy and safety of these medications in the treatment of xerostomia, thus their use is limited [13].

Salivary Substitutes

Water is commonly used as a salivary substitute however it provides short term relief and does not moisten or lubricate the oral mucosa and teeth adequately [1, 13]. The various salivary substitute agents that have been developed are based on carboxymethycellulose (CMC), xanthan gum and lactoperoxidase [3]. Other thickening agents include polyethylenoxide, polyacrylic acid and linseed polysaccharide extracts [13]. Agents containing polyacrylic acid are recommended in patients with extremely low salivary flow rates [13]. Although these agents provide symptomatic relief they do not completely replace the protective effects of saliva [3]. One commonly used salivary substitute is Biotene®. It is available as a sugar-free chewing gum and as an alcohol-free mouthwash and toothpaste [1]. It contains multiple enzymes that help maintain the healthy balance of oral flora [51]. In a phase II study conducted by Warde et al Biotene® was shown to improve visual analogue scale (VAS) scores (>10mm) in 54% of pateints with postradiation xerostomia [51]. Of those, 36% had major (>25mm) improvement in VAS scores [51]. In a double blind, crossover study Biotene® was compared with BioXtra in the treatment of postradiation xerostomia. Both products demonstrated a significant (p<0.05) improvement in VAS scores [52]. In a randomized control trial conducted by Femiano et al patients with drug induced xerostomia were given one of three types of mouthwash [53]. Group 1 received a salivary substitute solution (containing water, hydroxypropyl cellulose, sorbitol, dipotassium chloride, sodium chloride, magnesium chloride, calcium chloride and potassium phosphate). Group 2 recived a solution of citric acid (3% in essential water) and Group 3 received distilled water. At 15 minutes after administration both the salivary substitute and citric acid solution resulted in significantly reduced oral dryness ($p<0.001$). These results persisted at 1 hour post administration however the citric acid solution was more effective than the salivary substitute solution ($p=0.0047$) [53]. Despite the positive effects there are a variety of opinions regarding the use of salivary substitutes in the treatment of xerostomia. This discrepancy may be due to two major reasons: 1) efficacy of saliva substitutes are based on instruction given and the expectations of the patient and 2) the composition of commercially available saliva substitutes often differs from the substitutes tested in clinical trials [13]. The American Society of Clinical Oncology (ASCO) recommends using oral mucosal lubricants and salivary substitutes for the short-term improvement of xerostomia following radiotherapy as listed in their practice guidelines [7].

Treatment of Underlying Disorders

Treatment of the underlying disorder is the key in controlling xerostomia related to autoimmune dysfunction. Prednisone and perioxicam are often used in the treatment of Sjogren's however studies have not shown significant improvement in functional or histological parameters of the salivary and lacrimal glands [13]. Hydroxychloroquine has shown subjective improvement in oral symptoms (pain and dryness) in about sixty percent of patients and significantly increased salivary flow rate in 82 percent of patients [13]. Cyclosporin A, a T cell intervening treatment was shown to improve xerostomia symptoms in 88 percent of patients ($p<0.01$) but there was no effect on salivary and lacrimal gland function [13]. At a dose of 0.2 mg/kg/week methotrexate has been shown to improve symptoms of dry mouth and dry eyes [13].

Acupuncture

Acupuncture has been performed clinically to treat xerostomia. The underlying mechanism of how acupuncture affects salivary hypofunction is unclear; however it is likely multifactorial including stimulation of both the central and peripheral nervous system [2, 3, 54]. In looking at traditional Chinese medicine, the improvement in "Chi" in one or more of the 12 main meridians is hypothesized to stimulate saliva production [54]. Based on the theories of western medicine acupuncture is thought to activate the visceral sensory afferent and motor efferent neurons which increases blood flow to salivary glands. This neuronal and vascular activation subsequently increases blood flow which is the likely mechanism of salivary gland regeneration [2, 18, 54]. Auricular acupuncture may specifically activate the parasympathetic nervous system with a subsequent increase in salivary gland flow [18, 54, 55]. Other possible mechanisms include the stimulation of minor salivary glands present in non-irradiated buccal mucosa which leads to increased salivary production and improved mucosal moisture [56]. Studies by Dawidson et al have shown that acupuncture can stimulate an increased release of calcitonin gene-related peptide and vasoactive intestinal polypeptide which may positively affect the salivary flow rates of xerostomic patients [55, 57]. Acupuncture has been noted to increase the unstimulated salivary flow rates after 12-24 weeks of treatment [2, 3]. Contrary to previous studies, Homb et al demonstrated that in patient's receiving combination acupuncture (manual, auricular, electro-acupuncture) whole salivary flow rates, as measured by the Modified Schirmer's tests (MST), improved 42 percent in the first six weeks of treatment [54]. Electro-acupuncture is thought to intensify the effect of salivary production by increasing local blood flow [58].

The most efficient acupuncture treatment points and number of treatments have not yet been established however there have been reports of symptom relief in as little as five treatments [18, 28, 59]. Approaches can include manual, auricular or electro-acupuncture [18]. Studies utilizing methods that combine acupuncture and electrical stimulation have resulted in significant improvements in reported xerostomia and salivary flow rates (both stimulated and unstimulated) [56]. Studies utilizing combination acupuncture have demonstrated a greater than 30 percent increase in salivation, corresponding to a functional improvement in daily life and benefits from the treatment lasting up to 6 months [18, 54]. Until recently there has been no evidence supporting the effect of acupuncture on QOL; however in 2014 Homb et al published a retrospective case series of 16 patients that demonstrated combination acupuncture could significantly improve dry mouth, pain and sleep within the first 6 months of treatment [54]. He also demonstrated an improvement in swallowing, speaking and dry mouth with eating however change in taste did not show a specific trend [54]. The positive effects of acupuncture are only seen when residual salivary gland tissue remains functional and thus the success of the treatment depends on the degree of surgical excision and the size of the irradiated area [3]. Other positive effects of acupuncture include patient reported decrease in the viscosity of their saliva, improved taste, reduction of pain in the tongue and improvement of nausea and appetite [3]. The positive effects of acupuncture have been noted to last for 6 months and up to 3 years with additional acupuncture treatments [3]. Randomized control trials have demonstrated acupuncture to be a beneficial treatment in patients with radiation induced xerostomia who have already received IMRT [28, 60]. Three components typically contribute to the effects of acupuncture: a non-specific placebo effect, related to the patient's expectation and relationship with the acupuncturist; physiological effect due to needles being inserted into the skin; and specific effect due to needling manipulation at specific acupoints [61, 62]. In addition to its reported symptom benefit, acupuncture is a cost-effective, minimally invasive, low risk procedure [28, 61].

Although there is documented benefit of the use of acupuncture in xerostomia there are many issues that still remain. Standardized methods of evaluating and comparing the efficacy of acupuncture are needed. Salivary flow if often used as an outcome measure however there are varying methods of measurement and thus comparisons between studies are suboptimal [61]. Most importantly, placebo-controlled trials are needed to clearly investigate the short and long term clinical effects of acupuncture in xerostomic patients; determine the efficacy of prevention and treatment of xerostomia and to delineate specific treatment guidelines [61]. The ASCO suggests the use of acupuncture to stimulate salivary gland secretion and to alleviate xerostomia (Level II evidence, grade C recommendation) [7].

Hyperbaric Oxygen Therapy (HBOT)

HBOT is a system used to delivery oxygen to hypoxic tissues. It is frequently used to treat osteoradionecrosis of the mandible; however there are a few studies that have looked at its effect on radiation-induced tissue damage [3]. When administered immediately after radiotherapy, HBOT has been shown to improve xerostomia associated QOL as well as oral functions such as eating [24]. A study by Teguh et al. demonstrated significant improvement in 'sticky saliva' (p=0.01) and 'dry mouth items' (p=0.009) and also noted no oral pain at 6 weeks after treatment (p=0.011) [6]. HBOT has also been shown to demonstrate a statistically significant increase in salivary flow 1 to 2 years after treatment [3]. The direct mechanism of how HBOT improves salivary hypofunction is not known but it is understood that HBOT provides long term effects on neovascularization, osteoneogenesis, stimulation of collagen formation and improvement in wound healing due to mobilization of stem cells all of which may contributes to its effects on hyposalivation [3, 24]. The current literature reports inconsistent data regarding the use of this treatment in xerostomia thus there is a need for further studies to clearly delineate the role of HBOT in the treatment of radiation induced xerostomia [6]. At present there are no recommendations for the use of HBOT for the treatment of radiation induced xerostomia (Level IV evidence, grade D recommendation) [63].

Stimulants

Salivary secretion is mostly controlled the parasympathetic nervous system thus one of the most productive ways to combat xerostomia is to stimulate the salivary gland receptors [1]. This stimulation can be accomplished by both physiological and pharmacological means [1]. It has been noted that reduced mastication can exacerbate atrophy of the salivary glands [64] thus research has indicated the important of physiological stimulation of these glands by either masticatory or gustatory stimuli [1]. Methods of stimulating the glands include xylitol chewing gum, sucking sugar-free or acidic candies and stimulating lozenges [3, 4, 44, 65]. Research has demonstrated that these non-pharmacological agents that have demonstrated an increase in whole saliva secretion and an improvement in oral dryness [66, 67]. This improvement is mainly due to a) the act of chewing itself is associated with enhanced salivation through effects on oral baroreceptors and b) stimulation of the taste receptors may also contribute to enhanced salivary response [1].

An alternative treatment that has been studied for the treatment of xerostomia is electrical stimulation (E-stim). This is a treatment based on theory of acupuncture. It utilizes high-intensity and low frequency noninvasive transcutaneous electrical nerve stimulation (TENS) that activates A-beta and suppresses A-delta and C nerve fibers [3]. This mechanism mimics the sensation of acupuncture however it does not require the use of invasive needles nor does it require the expertise required for acupuncture treatment [56, 68, 69]. Despite the fact that there is little literature that supports this non-pharmacological treatment approach, there are some studies that have shown a statistically significant improvement in visual analog scale (VAS) scores for xerostomia symptoms in patients being treated for HNC radiation [56]. The VAS utilized in this phase I-II study consisted of five questions that assessed the dryness of the patient's mouth. Each item was set up with the most negative response (ie-the worst symptom or zero score) as the left anchor and the most positive response (ie-the absence of the symptom or score of 100) as the right anchor. Patients were instructed to mark their response on the scale relative to the two extremes with a higher score indicating the symptom was better controlled or absent. There is no known effect of E-stim on QOL scores [3]. A specific electrostimulation device that has been studied is called the GenNario, an intraoral device that delivers low intensity electrical current in the area of the lingual nerve [70]. The device was studied in patients who had xerostomia of varying etiologies (SS, radiotherapy, medications, graft versus host disease and idiopathic). Patients averaged 18 minutes of device use per day for 11 months [70]. Outcome measurements included xerostomia severity (as assessed by a questionnaire), QOL and resting and stimulated salivary flow rate. Except for QOL, all outcome variables (xerostomia severity including dryness severity, frequency of dryness, oral discomfort, speech, swallowing and sleep; resting salivary flow rate and stimulated salivary flow rate) showed positive results at the end of the 11 month period [70]. Based on the results of this study electrostimulation appears to be a safe, minimal risk treatment approach to xerostomia of varying etiologies [70].

Gene Transfer/Therapy

The role of gene transfer in the treatment of radiation induced hyposalivation is still in the early phase. Currently there are no clinical studies on human salivary glands. Studies conducted in rats and miniature pigs have been examining the transfer of human aquaporin-1 (hAQP1) cDNA. This aquaporin encodes a water channel that allows the movement of water along an osmotic gradient and subsequently could increase fluid to irradiated glands [3]. Preliminary studies have shown transient results lasting 2-4 weeks however these studies have led to the development of phase I/II clinical trial that is currently underway [71, 72].

Stem Cell Replacement

Many treatment options require the presence of residual gland tissue however tissue sparing is not always possible thus stem cell replacement has become a topic of research in the treatment of radiation induced hyposalivation [3]. Initial animal studies have shown that when transplanted in irradiated human salivary glands, murine stem cells have the ability to restore function and morphology [73]. In a later study conducted by Feng et al. it was discovered that human salivary glands contain stem cell populations that are similar to murine glands thus suggesting the potential to develop human stem cell therapy [74]. Further human studies are needed to further delineate this possibility.

Oral Care

Dental decay, cavities and gingivitis are common complications in those with xerostomia thus regular dental visits, at least three times per year, are important to maintaining appropriate oral hygiene [4]. Oral care products without alcohol are best utilized in the setting of xerostomia as alcohol can cause further drying of the oral mucosa [4]. Other important criteria in oral care products include those with a low pH, sugar-free, non-acidic and have added lubricants [4]. Oral care products containing xylitol are safe to use in xerostomia as it has been shown to have anti-caries properties [4].

Dry mouth places patients at a higher risk of fungal infections due to their reduced salivary flow and concomitant reduced mechanical cleansing [4, 13]. Changes in salivary composition can also reduce the natural inhibition of bacterial growth in the oral cavity which subsequently leads to an increase in caries-forming microbes and possibly bone infections [28]. Those with xerostomia who wear removable dentures are at an even higher risk of fungal infections and in the setting of candidiasis they should clean their dentures with chlorhexidine 1% gel twice daily [13]. Treatment of oral candidiasis, mostly angular cheilitis (19-35%) and acute erythematous candidiasis (38-65%) consists of miconazole 2% gel four times daily for at least two weeks [13]. Refractory cases may require the use of amphotericin B lozenges (10mg) four times daily for at least two weeks [13]. Patients should be advised that consumption of sugar free yogurt with active yeast cultures can help control oral fungal infections and to use antifungal agents without flavoring as this unnecessarily adds sugar [4].

Other

A number of different approaches targeted at biologic pathways have been attempted to try to modify the underlying autoimmunity, primarily in Sjogren's syndrome, contributing to the salivary gland dysfunction [4]. Interferon alpha dosed orally at 150-450 international units (IU) three times a day, has been shown to increase the stimulated whole salivary flow rates at 12 weeks compared to placebo however there was no significant difference at 24 weeks when compared to placebo [4]. Anti-Tumor necrosis factor alpha (TNFα) agents have been studied in the treatment of xerostomia however Infliximab, Entanercept and Thalidomide have not shown significant efficacy in randomized controlled trials involving patients with Sjogren's syndrome [4]. As there is well documented B-cell hyperactivity in Sjogren's syndrome, interest has been placed at modulation of B cell activation. In an open label study using Rituximab, a monoclonal antibody that binds to the CD20 antigen, there were documented improvements in symptoms of dry mouth and salivary gland function [4]. Despite these findings, a randomized control trial is needed prior to recommendation of this treatment in Sjogren's syndrome related xerostomia.

Patients with symptoms of xerostomia should avoid caffeine intake and cigarette smoking due to their drying and irritating effects on the oral mucosa [4]. Home remedies that can be attempted include a room humidifier and oral lubricants such as vegetable oil [4, 13].

Although salivary gland dysfunction is irreversible, preventative measures and conservative treatments can avoid or limit mucosal breakdown, infections and permanent damage to teeth [4]. Adequate symptom relief and increasing salivary flow is important as it may help patients feel more comfortable and improve their QOL [4]. Table 4 summarizes the treatment options.

Table 4. Treatment of xerostomia

Treatment	Trial type/results (Reference)
Pharmacological	
Pilocarpine	RCT/ Improved unstimulated saliva, p<0.001 (LeVeque 1993)
	RCT/ Improved whole(p=0.003) & unstimulated(p<0.001) saliva (Rieke 1995)
Cevimeline	RCT/ Improved unstimulated saliva, p=0.0068 (Petrone 2002)
Prednisone*	Double blind RCT/no effect (#27 from3)
Piroxicam*	Double blind RCT/no effect (#27 from 3)
Hydroxychloroquine*	Double blind, placebo controlled crossover/ no effect on salivary function (#38 from3)
	Open, retrospective/ improved salivary flow rate (#39 from 3)
Cyclosporin A*	Open (continuation of double blind study)/ improved xerostomia symptoms, p<0.01
	No effect on salivary gland function (29 from 3)
Methotrexate*	Open/ subjective improvement, no change in salivary gland function (#34 from 3)
(*these medications were tested for the treatment of xerostomia secondary to Sjogren syndrome)	
Salivary substitutes	
Biotene®	Double blind, crossover with BioXtra/both improved VAS scores, p<0.05 (Shahdad 2005)
	Phase II study/36% of patients had >25mm improvement in VAS scores (Warde 2000)
Citric Acid solution	RCT/ improved oral dryness, p=0.0047. no change in unstimulated saliva (Femiano 2011)
**The ASCO recommends the use of oral mucosal lubricants and salivary substitutes for the short-term improvement of radiation induced xerostomia	
Acupuncture	
	RCT/ improved unstimulated & stimulated salivary flow rates at 3 weeks (p=0.03),
	1 month & 6 months (p<0.0001) after radiotherapy (8)
Hyperbaric Oxygen Therapy	
	Randomized/ subjective improvement in 'sticky saliva' (p=0.01) and 'dry mouth
	(p=0.009) questionnaire items, no changes in oral pain (p=0.011) (Teguh 2009)
Salivary Stimulants	
(All studies listed were investigating the treatment of radiation induced xerostomia)	
Acidic candies	Prospective study/ increased whole saliva (#51 from13)
	Pilot study/ improved oral dryness and comfort (#50 from 13)
Electrical Stimulation	
GenNario	Multi-center, open label, uncontrolled clinical trial/ improved resting (p<0.001) and stimulated salivary flow (p<0.02) (9)
Gene Transfer/Therapy	
	Preliminary animal studies/ transient increase in salivary flow (#59 from 13)
Stem Cell	(Phase I/II clinical trials are currently underway)
	Animal studies/ murine stem cells were able to restore function when transplanted into human salivary glands (#65 from13)
	Animal & human tissue study/ human salivary glands contain stem cell populations similar to murine glands (#66 from 13)

Conclusion

Xerostomia is a symptom caused by multiple etiologies including polypharmacy, radiation or chemoradiation of head and neck cancer, systemic disorders and autoimmune diseases. Its association with impaired swallowing/speech, altered tasted, sleep disturbance and poor nutrition can have a significant impact on a patient's quality of life. Due to these effects it is a condition that clinicians should be aware of in order to help institute preventative measures and ameliorate oral complications [4]. A variety of available options are summarized in this article to facilitate the clinical prevention and treatment of xerostomia. Given the lack of specific guidelines in the management of xerostomia there is a need for a universal tool to evaluate radiation induced hyposalivation and the consequent xerostomia [3]. However, the difficulty in developing an evaluation tool lies in the fact that there are no specific criteria or threshold at which salivary gland dysfunction correlates to a patient's reported symptoms [4]. Research, particularly randomized trials, would help provide the optimal options to prevent and treat xerostomia in the future [3].

References

[1] Cassolato, SF and Turnbull RS. Xerostomia: Clinical Aspects and Treatment. *Gerodontology*. 2003. Dec; 20(2): 64-77.

[2] Bhide SA, Miah B, Harrington KJ, Newbold KL, Nutting CM. Radiation-induced Xerostomia: Pathophysiology, Prevention and Treatment. *Clinical Oncology* (2009) 21: 737-744.

[3] Lovelace TL, Fox NF, Sood AJ, Nguyen SA, Day TA. Management of radiotherapy-induced salivary hypofunction and consequent xerostomia in patinets with oral or head and neck cancer: meta-analysis and literature review. *Oral Surg. Oral Med. Oral Pathol. Oral Radiol.* 2014 May; 117(5): 595-607.

[4] Fox PC. Xerostomia: Recognition and Management. Dent Assist. 2008 Sept-Oct; 77(5): 18,20, 44-8; quiz 50-1.

[5] Bartels CL. Xerostomia. http://www.oralcancerfoundation.org/complications/xero stomia.php

[6] Teguh DN, Levendage PC, Noever I et al. Early Hyperbaric Oxygen Therapy For Reducing Radiotherapy Side Effects: Early Results of A Randomized Trial in Oropharyngeal And Nasopharyngeal Cancer. *Int. J. Radiation Oncology Biol. Phys.* 2009; 75:711-6.

[7] Kaluzny J, Wierzbicka M, Nogala H, Milecki P, Kopec T. Radiotherapy induced xerostomia: Mechanisms, diagnostics, prevention and treatment- Evidence based up to 2013. *Otolaryngologia Polska* 68 (2014). 1-14.

[8] Shaha AR, Patel S, Shasha D, Harrison LB. Head and Neck Cancer. In: LenhardREJr, Osteen RT, GanslerT, editors. Clinical Oncology. Atlanta Ga: American Cancer Society; 2001. P 297-330.

[9] Criswell MA, Sinha CK. Hyperthermic, supersaturated humidification in the treatment of xerostomia. *Laryngoscope* 2001; 111: 992-996.

[10] Logemann JA, Smith CH, Pauloski BR et al. Effects of xerostomia on perception and performance of swallow function. *Head Neck* 2001; 23: 317-321.

[11] Chambers MS, Toth BB, Martin JW, Fleming TJ, Lemon JC. Oral and dental management of the cancer patient; prevention and treatment of complications. *Support Care Cancer* 1995; 3: 168-175.

[12] Spielman AI. Interaction of saliva and taste. *J. Dent. Res.* 1990; 69: 838-843.

[13] van der Reijden WA, Vissink A, Veerman ECI, Nieuw Amerongen AV. Treatment of oral dryness related complaints (xerostomia) in Sjogren's syndrome. *Ann. Rheum. Dis.* 1999; 58: 465-473.

[14] Liu B, Dion MR, Jurasic MM, Gibson G, Jones J. Xerostomia and salivary gland hypofunction in vulnerable elders: prevalence and etiology. *Oral Medicine.* Vol 114. No. 1. July 2012.

[15] Wong HM. Oral Complications and Management Strategies for Patients Undergoing Cancer Therapy. *ScientificWorldJournal.* 2014.

[16] Caribe-Gomes F, Chimenos-Kustner E, Lopez-Lopez J et al. Dental management of the complications of radio and chemotherapy in oral cancer. *Med. Oral* 2003; 8: 178-187.

[17] Sreebny LM, Schwartz SS. A reference guide to drugs and dry mouth- 2nd edition. *Gerodontology* 1997: 14(1): 33-47.

[18] Wu H, Wong K, Wang D. Relief of Radiation-Induced Xerostomia With Acupuncture Treatment: A Case Presentation. *PM&R.* Vol. 3, 85-87. January 2011.

[19] van de Water TA, Bijl HP, Westerlaan HE, Langendijk JA. Delineation guidelines for organs at risk involved in radiation-induced salivary dysfunction and xerostomia. *Radiother. Oncol.* 2009; 93(3): 545-552.

[20] Hoebers F, Yu E, Eisbruch A et al. A Pragmatic Contouring Guideline for Salivary Gland Structures in Head and Neck Radiation Oncology. The MOIST Target. *American Journal of Clinical Oncology.* Vol. 36, Number 1, February 2013.

[21] Lee C, Langen KM, Lu W, Haimerl J, Schnarr E, Ruchala KJ et al. Evaluation of geometric changes of parotid glands during head and neck cancer radiotherapy using daily MVCT and automatic deformable registration. *Radiother. Oncol.* 2008; 89(1): 81-88.

[22] Eisbruch A, Kim HM, Terrell JE, Marsh LH, Dawson LA, Ship JA. Xerostomia and Its Predictors Following Parotid-Sparing Irradiation of Head and Neck Cancer. *Int. J. Radiation Oncology Biol. Phys.*, Vol. 50, No. 3, pp. 695-704, 2001.

[23] Chambers MS. Clinical commentary on prophylactic treatment of radiation-induced xerostomia. *Arch. Otolaryngol. Head Neck Surg.* 2003; 129:251-252.

[24] Porter SR. Fedele S. Habbab KM. Xerostomia in head and neck malignancy. *Oral Oncology* 46 (2010) 460-463.

[25] Gaubitz M. Epidemiology of connective tissue disorders. *Rheumatology*, 2006; 45.

[26] Usuba FS, Lopes JB, Fuller R, Yamamoto JH et al. Sjogren's syndrome: An underdiagnosed condition in mixed connective tissue disease. *Clinics.* 2014; 69 (3): 158-162.

[27] Pow EH, Kwong DL, McMillan AS et al. Xerostomia and Quality of Life After Intensity-Modulated Radiotherapy vs. Conventional Radiotherapy for Early-Stage Nasopharyngeal Carcinoma: Initial Report on a Randomized Controlled Clinical Trial. *Int. J. Radiation Oncology Biol. Phys.,* Vol 66, No 4, pp.981-991, 2006.

[28] Meng Z, Kay Garcia M, Hu C et al. Randomized Controlled Trial of Acupuncture for Prevention of Radiation-Induced Xerostomia Among Patients with Nasopharyngeal Carcinoma. *Cancer*. 2012; 118: 3337-44.

[29] Eisbruch A, Rhodus N, Rosenthal D et al. The prevention and treatment of radiotherapy-induced xerostomia. *Semin. Radiat. Oncol.* 2003; 13: 302-208.

[30] Amosson CM, The BS, Van TJ et al. Dosimetric predictors of xerostomia for head and neck cancer patients treated with the smart (simultaneous modulated accelerated radiation therapy) boost technique. *Int. J. Radiat. Oncol. Biol. Phys.* 2003; 56: 136-144.

[31] Eisbruch A, Ten H RK, Kim HM et al. Dose, volume, and function relationships in parotid salivary glands following conformal and intensity-modulated irradiation of head and neck cancer. *Int. J. Radiat. Oncol. Biol. Phys.* 1999; 45:577-587.

[32] Mendenhall WM, Amdur RJ, Palta JR. Intensity-modulated radiotherapy in the standard management of head and neck cancer: promises and pitfalls. *J. Clin. Oncol.* 2006; 24:2618-2623.

[33] Giatromanolaki A, Sivridis E, Maltezos E, Koukourakis MI. Down-regulation of intestinal-type alkaline phosphatase in the tumor vasculature and stroma provides a strong basis for explaining amifostine selectivity. *Semin. Oncol.* 2002; 29(6 Suppl 19): 14-21.

[34] Brizel, DM, Wasserman TH, Henke M, Strnad V et al. Phase III Randomized Trial of Amifostine as a Radioprotector in Head and Neck Cancer. *J. of Clin. Oncology*, Vol 18, No 19 (October 1), 2000: pp 3339-3345.

[35] Bardet E, Martin L, Calais G, Alfonsi M et al. Subcutaneous Compared with Intravenous Administration of Amifostine in Patients With Head and Neck Cancer Receiving Radiotherapy: Final Results of the GORTEC 2000-02 Phase III Randomized Trial. *J. of Clin. Oncology*, Vol 29, No 2 (January 10) 2011, pp 127-133.

[36] Zhang X, Liu F, Lan X, Yu L et al. Clinical observation of submandibular gland transfer for the prevention of xerostomia after radiotherapy for nasopharyngeal carcinoma: a prospective randomized controlled study of 32 cases. *Radiation Oncology* 2014, 9:62.

[37] Jha N, Seikaly H, McGaw T, Coulter L. Submandibular salivarygland transfer prevents radiation induced xerostomia. *Int. J. Radiat. Oncol. Biol. Phys.* 2000, 46: 7-11.

[38] Saibishkumar EP, Jha N, Scrimger RA, MacKenzie MA et al. Sparing the parotid glans and surgically transferred submandibular gland with helical tomotherapy in post-operative radiation of head and neck cancer: a planning study. *Radiother. Oncol.* 2007, 85: 98-104.

[39] Jha N, Seikaly H, Harris J, Williams D et al. Phase III randomized study: oral pilocarpine versus submandibular salivary gland transfer protocol for the management of radiation-induced xerostomia. *Head Neck* 2009, 31: 234-243.

[40] Seikaly H, Jha N, McGawT, Coulter L et al. Submandibular gland transfer: a new method of prevention radiation- induced xerostomia. *Laryngoscope* 2001, 111:347-352.

[41] Teymoortash A, Muller F, Juricko J, Bieker M et al. Botulinum toxin prevents radiotherapy-induced salivary gland damage. *Oral Oncol.* 2009; 45(8): 737-739.

[42] Fox PC. Management of dry mouth. *Dent. Clin. North Am.* 1997; 41: 863-875.

[43] Garg AK, Malo M. Manifestations and treatment of xerostomia and associate oral effects secondary to head and neck radiation therapy. *J. Am. Dent. Assoc.* 1997; 128: 1128-1133.

[44] Odusola F. chewing gum as an aid in treatment of hyhposalivation. *NY State Dent. J.* 1991; 57: 28-31.

[45] LeVeque FG, Montgomery M, Potter D, Zimmer MB et al. A Multicenter, Randomized, Double-Blind, Placebo-Controlled, Dose-Titration Study of Oral Pilocarpine for Treatment of Radiation-Induced Xerostomia in Head and Neck Cancer Patients. *J. of Clin. Oncology*, Vol 11, No 6 (June), 1993: pp 1124-1131.

[46] Rieke JW, Hafermann MD, Johnson JT, LeVeque FG et al. Oral Pilocarpine For Radiation-Induced Xerostomia: Integrated Efficacy And Safety Results From Two Prospective Randomized Clinical Trials. *Int. J. Radiation Oncology Biol. Phys.*, Vol. 31, No. 3, pp. 661-669, 1995.

[47] Ringash J, Warde P, Lockwood G, O'Sullivan B et al. Postradiotherapy quality of life for head-and-neck cancer patients is independent of xerostomia. *Int. J. Radiat. Oncol. Biol. Phys*, 2005; 61(5): 1403-1407.

[48] Warde P, O'Sullivan B, Aslanidis J, Kroll B et al. A Phase III Placebo-Controlled Trial of Oral Pilocarpine in Patients Undergoing Radiotherapy for Head-and-Neck Cancer. *Int. J. Radiat. Oncol. Biol. Phys*, 2002; 54(1): 9-13.

[49] Petrone D, Condemi JJ, Fife R, Gluck O et al. A Double-Blind, Randomized, Placebo-Controlled Study of Cevimeline in Sjoren's Syndrome Patinets with Xerostomia and Keratoconjunctivitis Sicca. *Arthritis & Rheumatism.* Vol. 46, No. 3, March 2002, pp 848-754.

[50] Chambers MS, Garden AS, Kies MS, Martin JW. Radiation-induced xerostomia in patients with head and neck cancer: pathogenesis, impact, quality of life, and management. *Head Neck* 2004; 26(9): 796-807.

[51] Warde P, Kroll B, O'Sullivan B et al. A phase II study of Biotene in the treatment of postradiation xerostomia in patients with head and neck cancer. *Support Care Cancer* 2000; 8:203-208.

[52] Shahadad SA, Taylor C, Barclay SC, Steen LN et al. A double-blind, crossover study of Biotene Oralbalance and BioXtra systems as salivary substitutes in patients with post-radiotherapy xerostomia. *European Journal of Cancer Care* 2005, 14, 319-326.

[53] Femiano F, Rullo R, diSpirito F, Lanza A et al. A comparison of salivary substitutes versus a natural sialogogue (citric acid) in patients complaining of dry mouth as an adverse drug reaction: a clinical, randomized controlled study. *Oral Surg. Oral Med. Oral Pathol. Oral Radiol. Endod.* 2011; 112: e15-e20.

[54] Homb KA, Wu H, Tarima S, Wang D. Improvement of radiation-induced xerostomia with acupuncture: A retrospective analysis. *Acupuncture Relat. Ther.* (2014), pp 34-38.

[55] Dawidson I, Angmar-Mansson B, Blom M, Theodorsson E et al. Sensory stimulation (acupuncture) increases the release of calcitonin gene-related peptide in the saliva of xerostomia sufferers. *Neuropeptides* 1999; 33: 244-250.

[56] Wong RK, Jones GW, Sagar SM, Babjak AF et al. A phase I-II study in the use of acupuncture-like transcutaneous nerve stimulation in the treatment of radiation-induced xerostomia in head-and-neck cancer patients treated with radical radiotherapy. *Int. J. Radiat. Oncol. Biol. Phys.* 2003; 57(2): 472-480.

[57] Dawidson I, Angmar-Mansson B, Blom M, Theodorsson E et al Sensory stimulation (acupuncture) increases the release of vasoactive intestinal polypeptide in the saliva of xerostomia sufferers. *Neuropeptides*. 1998; 32: 543-548.

[58] Blom M, Lundeberg T, Dawidson I, Angmar-Mansson B. Effects on local blood flux of acupuncture stimulation used to treat xerostomia in patients suffereing from Sjogren's syndrome. *J. Oral Rehab.* 2007; 20: 541-548.

[59] Rydholm M, Strang P. Acupuncture for patients in hospital-based home care suffering from xerostomia. *J. Palliat. Care.* 1999; 15: 20-23.

[60] Garcia MK, Chiang JS, Cohen L et al. Acupuncture for radiation-induced xerostomia in patients with cancer: a pilot study. *Head Neck.* 2009; 31: 1360-1368.

[61] Zhuang L, Yang Z, Zeng X, Zhua X, et al. The Preventative and Therapeutic Effect of Acupuncture for Radiation-Induced Xerostomia in Patients With Head and Neck Cancer: A Systematic Review. *Integrative Cancer Therapies.* 2012. 12(3), 197-205.

[62] White AR, Filshie J, Cummings TM. Clinical trials of acupuncture: consensus recommendations for optimal treatment, sham controls and blinding. *Complement. Ther. Med.* 2001; 9: 237-245.

[63] Gerlach NL, Barkhuysen R, Kaanders JH, Janssens GO, et al. The effect of hyperbaric oxygen therapy on quality of life in oral and oropharyngeal cancer patients treated with radiotherapy. *Int. J. Oral Maxillofac. Surg.* 2008; 37(3): 255-259.

[64] Atkinson JL, Wu AJ. Salivary gland dysfunction: causes, symptoms and treatment. *J. Am. Dent. Assoc.* 1994; 125: 409-416.

[65] Daniels TE, Wu AJ. Xerostomia- clinical evaluation and treatment in general practice. *J. Can. Dent. Assoc.* 2000; 28: 933-941.

[66] Sanahayake F, Piggott K, Hamilton-Miller JM. A pilot study of Salix SST (saliva-stimulating lozenges) in post-irradiation xerostomia. *Curr. Med. Res. Opin.* 1998: 14(3): 155-159.

[67] Jensdottir T, Nauntofte B, Buchwald C, Hansen HS, et al. Effects of sucking acidic candies on saliva in unilaterally irradiated pharyngeal cancer patients. *Oral Oncol.* 2006; 42(3): 317-322.

[68] Wong RK, Sagar SM, Chem BJ, Yi GY, et al. Phase II randomized trial of acupuncture-like transcutaneous electrical nerve stimulation to prevent radiation-induced xerostomia in head and neck cancer patinets. *J. Soc. Integr. Oncol.* 2010; 8:35-42.

[69] Wong RK, James JL, Sagar S, et al. Phase 2 results from Radiation Therapy Oncology Group Study 0537: a phase 2/3 study comparing acupuncture-like transcutaneous electrical nerve stimulation versus pilocarpine in treating early radiation-induced xerostomia. *Cancer.* 2012; 118: 4244-4252.

[70] Alajbeg I, Falcao DP, Tran SD, Martin-Granizo R, et al. Intraoral electrostimulator for xerostomia relief: a long-term, multicenter, open-label, uncontrolled, clinical trial. *Oral Surg. Oral Med. Oral Pathol. Oral Radiol.* 2012 Jun; 113(6): 773-81.

[71] Zheng C, Goldsmith CM, Mineshiba F, et al. Toxicity and biodistribution of a first-generation recombinant adenoviral vector, encoding aquaporin-1, after retroductal delivery to a single rat submandibular gland. *Hum. Gene Ther.* 2006; 17: 1122-1133.

[72] Baum BJ, Zheng C, Alevizos I, et al. Development of a gene transfer-baed treatment for radiation-induced salivary hypofunction. *Oral Oncol.* 2010; 46: 4-8.

[73] Lombaert IM, Brunsting JF, Wierenga PK, et al. Rescus of slivary gland function after stem cell transplantation in irradiated glands. *PLoS One.* 2008; 3:e2063.

[74] Feng J, van der Zwaag M, Stokman MA, va Os R, et al. Isolation and characterization of human salivary gland cells for stem cell transplantation to reduce radiation-induced hyposalivation. *Radiother. Oncol.* 2009: 92: 466-471.

In: Horizons in Cancer Research. Volume 55
Editor: Hiroto S. Watanabe

ISBN: 978-1-63463-228-7
© 2015 Nova Science Publishers, Inc.

Chapter 5

Causes of Xerostomia in the Cancer Treatment

Eliana Aparecida Minicucci[1],*,
Silke Anna Theresa Weber[2]
and Glenda Nicioli da Silva[3]

[1]UNESP – Universidade Estadual Paulista; Botucatu Medical School;
Department of Dermatology and Radiotherapy – Botucatu – SP – Brazil
[2]UNESP – Universidade Estadual Paulista; Botucatu Medical School;
Department of Ophthalmology and Otolaryngology - Botucatu - SP, Brazil
[3]UFOP – Universidade Federal de Ouro Preto; Pharmacy School;
Department of Clinical Analysis – Ouro Preto – MG – Brazil

Abstract

Saliva is fundamental for the maintenance of oral health. It is a complex mix of fluids secreted by major and minor salivary glands. Xerostomia is the subjective sensation of dry mouth, that can be associated or not to the diminution of the salivary flow. It predominantly affects middle aged and elderly people with an estimated prevalence of 21% and 27% in men and women, respectively. Oral dryness can profoundly affect the quality of life, interfering to basic daily functions such as chewing, swallowing and speaking. Reduction of volume and the antibacterial properties of saliva may cause infections, accelerate tooth decay and periodontal disease. The most important causes of xerostomia include factors that act on the salivary center in the central nervous system related to emotions; the autonomic nervous system caused by encephalitis, cerebral tumors, cerebral vascular accidents, neurosurgery or drugs; autoimmune disease, viral or bacteria salivary gland infections, radiotherapy and chemotherapy and the hydro–electrolytic balance related to cystic fibrosis, primary cirrhoses, sarcoidosis, amyloidosis, hypothireoidism and hemochromatosis. The oral epithelium has a high "turn over", therefore is one of the main places in which manifest the side effects of chemotherapy

* Corresponding author: eminicucci@hotmail.com.

(CT) and head and neck radiotherapy (RT). The xerostomia caused by RT can be due to indirect damage to epithelial and connective tissue elements of the gland, or direct damage to salivary acini and ducts. High-dose chemotherapy may affect the salivary flow, principally in hematopoietic cell transplantation, total body irradiation and concurrent medications.

Abbreviations

RT	radiotherapy
CT	chemotherapy
IMRT	intensity modulated radiation therapy
GVHD	chronic graft-versus-host disease
HCT	hematopoietic cell transplantation

Saliva

Saliva is fundamental for the maintenance of oral health, therefore deficits in the amount and quality of the gland secretions can exert negative effects upon oral mucosal health [1]. It is a complex mix of fluids secreted by major and minor salivary glands. It is characterized as a slightly acidic and clear mucoserosa exocrine secretion [2]. Most saliva volume is produced by the so called major saliva glands, as the parotid, submandibular and sublingual. The minor glands are located on the lips, tongue, hard and soft palate, buccal mucosa and pharynx and they are responsible for the production of protective compounds. The saliva is essential for a number of critical functions in the homeostasis of the oral ecosystem, in the oropharynx and larynx, and in speech and swallowing functions [3] facilitating the irrigation, lubrication and protection of the mucous membranes in the upper digestive tract [4].

Table 1. Salivary components and their functions [6, 8-10]

Components	Functions
Electrolytes	Maintain pH and buffering capacities
Immunoglobulins (IgA)	Inhibit microbial adherence
Mucins	Maintain lubrication of oral cavity protecting against infections
Glycoptotein, lisosyme, lactoferin	Antimicrobial action
Histatins	Antifungal action
Amylase, lipase, proteases, nucleases, mucins, gustin	Digestive process

The saliva is composed of water (99%) [5], inorganic ions Ca^{+2}, Mg^{+2}, K^+, Na^+, HCO_3^-, Cl^-, $H_3PO_4^-$, HPO_4^-, F^-, and others substances such as albumin, ammonia, amylase, creatinine, cystatins, esterases, glucose, gustin, histatins, immunoglobulins (IgA, IgG, IgM), iodine, kallikrein, lactoferrin, lactoperoxidase, lactic dehydrogenase, lysozyme, mucins, nitrogen, proline-rich proteins, ribonucleases, serum proteins, sialic acid statherin, sulfates, thiocyanate, and urea [2, 6-8]. The principal salivary components and their functions are described in table

1. The normal salivary pH is 6 to 7, and depends on the bicarbonate concentration. However, the pH can range from 5.3 (low-flow) to 7.8 (high flow) [2].

Salivary Flow

Total daily flow of whole saliva is, on average, between 500 mL and 1.5 L of unstimulated saliva (above 0.1mL/min) and 0.2mL/min for stimulated saliva [2]. The unstimulated salivary flow corresponds to 20% from parotid, 65% from submandibular, 7% to 8% from sublingual, and less than 10% from minor glands. In the stimulated salivary flow, there is a change in the contribution of each gland in the salivary flow, where the parotid contributing is more than 50% of total salivary secretions [11].

The salivary flow rate varies individually: daily (circadian) with low flow during sleep and peaks during high stimulation periods and annual (circannual) with low flow during the summer and peaks during the winter [11]. Circadian flow variations affect not only flow but also the concentration level of salivary components such as salivary electrolytes and proteins [12].

Saliva contains antimicrobial factors and growth factors that reduces the risk of mucosal trauma and promotes healing of damaged mucosa [13]. One of the most important functions of saliva is maintain the dental enamel integrity through of calcium and phosphate [14]. Saliva provides the first stage of the digestive process and in bolus formation and smooth transport during swallowing.

Diminished saliva increases the risk of caries, oral infections, mucositis, burning, tongue fissures, dysgeusia, halitosis, difficulty speaking, chewing and swallowing, resulting in impairment quality of life [15, 16].

Xerostomia is the subjective sensation of dry mouth that may be associated to the diminution of the salivary flow. It predominantly affects the middle aged and elderly people with an estimated prevalence of 21% and 27% in men and women, respectively [17]. The reduction of salivary flow by 40% to 50% is necessary for a patient to become symptomatic and develop xerostomia [18, 19]. The symptoms of xerostomia or dry mouth include dryness, burning sensation or discomfort, cracked lips, changes in the tongue surface, and problems in wearing removable dentures [20, 21]. Oral dryness can profoundly affect quality of life, interfering with basic daily functions such as chewing, swallowing, and speaking. Reduction of salivary volume and subsequent loss of the antibacterial properties of saliva may accelerate gengival and dental infections, tooth decay, and periodontal disease [18, 22-25].

Causes of xerostomia include factors that act: 1) on the salivary center caused by anxiety, fear, stress or depression, drugs of central action (opiaceous), cerebral tumors or Parkinson's diseases [26]; 2) on the autossomic system including encephalitis, cerebral tumors, cerebral vascular accident, neurosurgery or drugs [27]; 3) on the salivary gland function such as autoimmune disease, diffuse connective tissue diseases, viral or bacteria salivary gland infections, salivary gland tumors, radiotherapy and chemotherapy, diabetes mellitus, AIDS, or HCV infections [18, 24, 28]; 4) in less frequent, on the hydro – electrolytic balance including cystic fibrosis, primary cirrhoses, sarcoidosis, amyloidosis, hypothireoidism and hemochromatosis [18, 24].

Xerostomia in the Cancer Treatment

The oral complications of the cancer therapies result in acute and late toxicities. The acute oral complications include mucositis, infections, decreased of salivary flow and neurosensory change. Complications in survivors include neurosensory changes, xerostomia, taste alterations, functional changes, oral and dental infections, and risk of dental disease and necrosis of the jaw. The advances in cancer treatment have led to increased survival these patients and consequentely, changes in the incidence, nature, and severity of oral complications. Therefore, the management of late effects of cancer therapy are important for to improve the quality of life of these patients [3, 29].

Chemotherapy and radiotherapy are the main cancer treatment. The oral epithelium has a high "turn over", therefore is one of the main places in which manifest the side effects of chemotherapy (CT) and head and neck radiotherapy (RT).

Radiotherapy

The xerostomia is one of the principal late-effect of head and neck RT. The cervical region is main irradiated field in head and neck tumors, hitting directly or indirectly the major salivary glands such as parotid, submandibular and sublingual. The xerostomia caused by RT can be due to indirect damage to epithelial and connective tissue elements of the gland, or direct damage to salivary acini and ducts [30]. The direct damage may be related to p53-related apoptosis due to the development of reactive oxygen species leading to DNA damage and reduced insulin-like growth factor production [31, 32]. The salivary gland damage are related with dose and the volume of the gland irradiated [33]. Salivary tissue is sensitive with cumulative doses greater than 30 Gy, and can cause permanent salivary gland dysfunction that it is irreversible when the glands are within the RT field (33, 34). The serous acini (parotid gland) are more sensitive to RT resulting in decreased saliva volume and increased viscosity.

The early symptoms begin in the first weeks of RT with a decrease of about 50-60% of salivary flow with doses of 2 at 10 Gy [10], reaching a decrease of 90% of the total production of saliva [35-37]. In the end of the RT, the patients complain of thick saliva and impaired of oral clean. Usually this is caused by the drastic decrease in the volume of saliva produced by the parotid gland and increased concentration of mucin produced by the submandibular and sublingual glands. Depending of gland damage caused by RT, this late effect may persist for 6 months or to be irreversible [38-41].

The decreased salivary flow by RT may be cause dental demineralization and dental caries. These dental complications may be attributable to changes quantitative and qualitative of salivary compounds normally by decreased buffering capacity, calcium and phosphate, a shift in the oral flora to cariogenic bacteria (*Streptococcus mutans* and Lactobacillus sp.), [42, 43] and dietary changes [44, 45]. In most cases are pasty, which facilitates the accumulation of plaque, and this associated with a poor oral hygiene. The demineralization may progress to dental breakdown, periodontal disease and osteoradionecrosis [46].

The head and neck RT causes damage to taste buds and salivary glands resulting in reduced or loss taste sensibility that may improve in 8 weeks, several months after the RT

[47-53], and sometimes indefinitely, that may be due to damage to taste receptors [54]. Loss of taste is important because affects directly the diet and oral nutritional intake and it may have the strongest correlation with decreased quality of life in these patients [49].

The prevention of damage to the salivary glands is the most important in the control of xerostomia. This includes the use of 3-dimensional RT planning or IMRT, which provides more accurate distribution and optimization of the dose in the tumor volume and which saves the adjacent structures through the shaping and modulation of the radiation beam [10, 55-58]. The pharmacologic agents and surgical approaches have been evaluated to minimize salivary gland damage from RT [59-61].

Chemotherapy

CT is one of the most widely used management strategies in cancer, either alone or in combination with other types of treatment [62, 63]. The oral complications of CT are either a result of direct action of the drug upon the oral mucosa (direct stomatological toxicity), or an indirect consequence of chemotherapeutic drug-induced bone marrow suppression or myelosuppression (indirect stomatological toxicity, due principally the high cellular turnover rate of the oral mucosa [62, 63].

The drugs used in cancer therapy and in alleviation of symptoms related to cancer induce oral collateral effects, principally mucositis, hyposalivation, taste alterations [64] regardless of malignant tumor location. The oral late effects are related with the kind and dose of the CT drugs [64].

Salivary flow may be affected by high dose chemotherapy such as hematopoietic cell transplantation and bone marrow, chronic graft-versus-host disease (GVHD) due salivary gland involvement by GVHD and other drugs in combination [65, 66]. Inflammatory infiltration of the salivary glands and cytokine release causes an alteration in the quality of the saliva and reduces salivary quantity [3].

It was observed that the patients received chemotherapy for solid malignant tumors outside the head and neck region presented most notably xerostomia and mucositis in consequence of a high quantity of concurrent systemic medications [64]. Wilberg et al (2014) evaluated the oral health problems during chemotherapy in patients treated for solid tumors outside the head and neck region and observed that 59% of these patients presented xerostomia [64]. In a systematic review, the prevalence of xerostomia was observed in 50% of the patients during chemotherapy [67].

It has been observed a direct correlation between the degree of GVHD and salivary hypofunction: salivary fluid composition with higher salivary concentrations of sodium, magnesium, albumin, total protein, immunoglobulin (Ig) G, and epidermal growth factor and decreased IgA and inorganic phosphate, in addition to histopathological changes in the salivary gland [66]. In the chronic GVHD, the xerostomia can persist for months to years and occurs in 40% to 70% of surviving patients treated with allogeneic hematopoietic cell transplantation (HCT) from unrelated matched donors and in 25% to 45% of patients receiving allogeneic HCT from matched siblings [66]. Normally the xerostomia caused by CT is reversible, and the normal salivary flow returns in 2 to 3 months after the end of therapy [3].

The xerostomia treatment aim maintain the integrity of the oral mucosa but they are restricted to symptomatic therapy. The therapies include adequate oral hydration by the regular intake of water, oral hygiene with fluoride agents, antimicrobials to prevent dental caries, the use of cholinergic agonists such as pilocarpine, cevimeline or bethanechol, oral mucosa lubrificant/saliva substitutes for the patients not respond to pharmacological gustatory or masticatory stimulation [1, 68-70].

The therapies may improve the xerostomia, but generally the duration of relief is briefly. In the severe xerostomia is recommended a substitute with gel-like properties that may provide night-time relief, while a substitute with less viscous properties resembling natural saliva is recommended during the day [71]. Surgical transfer of the submandibular gland was described in the cases in that all major salivary glands are to be included in the RT field [47, 72-75]. Manual acupuncture using auricular points and, in some cases, supplemented with electro-stimulation has been described for providing relief from xerostomia [36, 76-78].

Taste disorders are common in cancer patients. It is estimated that 50-75% of cancer patients submitted chemotherapy, radiotherapy or both can presented alterations in taste perception and are related on the kind of cancer and its therapy [68]. In cancer patients, the main cause of dysgeusia is the action of chemotherapy and radiotherapy upon oral epithelial cell turnover, in addition to effects of such treatment upon nerves, taste buds and olfactory receptors [21, 63].

The flavor is based on four qualities: sweet, sour, salty and bitter. The taste is mediated by specialized epithelial cells distributed through the oral cavity, oropharynx, larynx, and upper esophagus. CT drugs can access the oral cavity through diffusion from plasma in the capillaries, producing an unpleasant taste [68, 79]. The dysgeusia also may be related to modifications in the concentrations of sodium, potassium and calcium in the taste bud cell receptors [79]. Other causes of taste disorders are candidiasis, viral infections, oral infection and oral hygiene, surgical, medications, head and neck RT, GVHD [80-82] and the hyposalivation due to limited delivery of taste to the receptors [83].

The taste alterations caused by chemotherapy is related to direct taste receptor stimulation due to secretion in saliva or via gingival crevice fluid. The patients frequently describe a metallic or chemical taste that can lead to dysgeusia and glossodynia secondary to the effects of chemotherapy upon the tongue papillae and demineralization of the nerve fibers [20, 21]. After of the drug clearance, the taste change may persist due to damage to the taste buds [20, 21, 84].

The dysgeusia therapy consist in the reduction of the dose of certain chemotherapeutic drugs (e.g., histone deacetylase inhibitors), the treatment of oral infections [68, 79], increased liquid intake during meals, chew food slowly, and especially increasing saliva production and pharmacological strategies such as zinc supplements and amifostine [68].

Final Conclusion

In conclusion, while there is evidence implicating the radiotherapy and chemotherapy in the important causes of xerostomia, some simple current therapies may improve the xerostomia, as the adequate oral hydration by the regular intake of water and the oral hygiene with fluoride agents antimicrobials to prevent dental caries and other. However, generally the duration of relief is briefly.

Thus, for minimize the risk of oral and systemic complications of cancer therapy is essential to evaluate the oral condition of the patient and treat all oral infections before cancer treatment [63, 85], improving the quality of life of these patients.

References

[1] Avsar A, Elli M, Darka O, Pinarli G. Long-term effects of chemotherapy on caries formation, dental development, and salivary factors in childhood cancer survivors. *Oral Surg. Oral Med. Oral Pathol. Oral Radiol Endod.* 2007 Dec; 104(6):781-9.

[2] Humphrey SP, Williamson RT. A review of saliva: normal composition, flow, and function. *J. Prosthet. Dent.* 2001 Feb; 85(2):162-9.

[3] Epstein JB, Thariat J, Bensadoun RJ, Barasch A, Murphy BA, Kolnick L, et al. Oral complications of cancer and cancer therapy: from cancer treatment to survivorship. *CA Cancer J. Clin.* 2012 Nov-Dec; 62(6):400-22.

[4] Guggenheimer J, Moore PA. Xerostomia: etiology, recognition and treatment. *J. Am. Dent. Assoc.* 2003 Jan; 134(1):61-9; quiz 118-9.

[5] Baum BJ. Neurotransmitter control of secretion. *J. Dent. Res.* 1987 Feb; 66 Spec No:628-32.

[6] Saliva: its role in health and disease. Working Group 10 of the Commission on Oral Health, Research and Epidemiology (CORE). *Int. Dent. J.* 1992 Aug; 42(4 Suppl 2):287-304.

[7] Fox PC. Saliva composition and its importance in dental health. *Compend. Suppl.* 1989(13): S457-60.

[8] Tenovuo J. Antimicrobial function of human saliva--how important is it for oral health? *Acta Odontol. Scand.* 1998 Oct; 56(5):250-6.

[9] Dowd FJ. Saliva and dental caries. *Dent. Clin. North Am.* 1999 Oct; 43(4):579-97.

[10] Santos PSS, Soares Junior LAVEsMBApnOHSP-SES, 2012. P287-303. Medicina Bucal. *A pratica na Odontologia Hospitalar.* São Paulo Editora Santos; 2012.

[11] Edgar WM. Saliva and dental health. Clinical implications of saliva: report of a consensus meeting. *Br. Dent. J.* 1990 Aug 11-25; 169(3-4): 96-8.

[12] Rudney JD. Does variability in salivary protein concentrations influence oral microbial ecology and oral health? *Crit. Rev. Oral. Biol. Med.* 1995; 6(4):343-67.

[13] Brosky ME. The role of saliva in oral health: strategies for prevention and management of xerostomia. *J. Support Oncol.* 2007 May; 5(5):215-25.

[14] Papas A, Russell D, Singh M, Kent R, Triol C, Winston A. Caries clinical trial of a remineralising toothpaste in radiation patients. *Gerodontology.* 2008 Jun; 25(2):76-88.

[15] Duncan GG, Epstein JB, Tu D, El Sayed S, Bezjak A, Ottaway J, et al. Quality of life, mucositis, and xerostomia from radiotherapy for head and neck cancers: a report from the NCIC CTG HN2 randomized trial of an antimicrobial lozenge to prevent mucositis. *Head Neck.* 2005 May; 27(5):421-8.

[16] Hopcraft MS, Tan C. Xerostomia: an update for clinicians. *Aust. Dent. J.* Sep; 55(3):238-44; quiz 353.

[17] Nederfors T, Isaksson R, Mornstad H, Dahlof C. Prevalence of perceived symptoms of dry mouth in an adult Swedish population--relation to age, sex and pharmacotherapy. *Community Dent. Oral Epidemiol.* 1997 Jun; 25(3):211-6.

[18] Al-Hashimi I. Xerostomia secondary to Sjogren's syndrome in the elderly: recognition and management. *Drugs Aging.* 2005; 22(11):887-99.

[19] Flink H, Tegelberg A, Lagerlof F. Influence of the time of measurement of unstimulated human whole saliva on the diagnosis of hyposalivation. *Arch. Oral Biol.* 2005 Jun; 50(6):553-9.

[20] Chan CW, Chang AM, Molassiotis A, Lee IY, Lee GC. Oral complications in Chinese cancer patients undergoing chemotherapy. *Support Care Cancer.* 2003 Jan; 11(1):48-55.

[21] Epstein JB, Tsang AH, Warkentin D, Ship JA. The role of salivary function in modulating chemotherapy-induced oropharyngeal mucositis: a review of the literature. *Oral Surg. Oral Med. Oral Pathol. Oral Radiol. Endod.* 2002 Jul; 94(1):39-44.

[22] Gupta A, Epstein JB, Sroussi H. Hyposalivation in elderly patients. *J. Can. Dent. Assoc.* 2006 Nov; 72(9):841-6.

[23] Amerongen AV, Veerman EC. Saliva--the defender of the oral cavity. *Oral Dis.* 2002 Jan; 8(1):12-22.

[24] Porter SR, Scully C, Hegarty AM. An update of the etiology and management of xerostomia. *Oral Surg. Oral Med. Oral Pathol. Oral Radiol. Endod.* 2004 Jan; 97(1):28-46.

[25] Fox RI, Liu AY. Sjogren's syndrome in dermatology. *Clin. Dermatol.* 2006 Sep-Oct; 24(5):393-413.

[26] Scully C. Drug effects on salivary glands: dry mouth. *Oral Dis.* 2003 Jul; 9(4):165-76.

[27] Teixeira MS, Weckx LLM. *Tratado de Otorrinolaringologia São Paulo:* Roca; 2003.

[28] Ship JA. Diagnosing, managing, and preventing salivary gland disorders. *Oral Dis.* 2002 Mar; 8(2):77-89.

[29] Jemal A, Siegel R, Xu J, Ward E. Cancer statistics, 2010. *CA Cancer J. Clin.* 2010 Sep-Oct; 60(5):277-300.

[30] Lin SC, Jen YM, Chang YC, Lin CC. Assessment of xerostomia and its impact on quality of life in head and neck cancer patients undergoing radiotherapy, and validation of the Taiwanese version of the xerostomia questionnaire. *J. Pain Symptom Manage.* 2008 Aug; 36(2):141-8.

[31] Grundmann O, Mitchell GC, Limesand KH. Sensitivity of salivary glands to radiation: from animal models to therapies. *J. Dent. Res.* 2009 Oct; 88(10):894-903.

[32] Limesand KH, Schwertfeger KL, Anderson SM. MDM2 is required for suppression of apoptosis by activated Akt1 in salivary acinar cells. *Mol. Cell Biol.* 2006 Dec; 26(23):8840-56.

[33] Murphy BA, Dietrich MS, Wells N, Dwyer K, Ridner SH, Silver HJ, et al. Reliability and validity of the Vanderbilt Head and Neck Symptom Survey: a tool to assess symptom burden in patients treated with chemoradiation. *Head Neck.* 2010 Jan; 32(1):26-37.

[34] Cassolato SF, Turnbull RS. Xerostomia: clinical aspects and treatment. *Gerodontology.* 2003 Dec; 20(2):64-77.

[35] Dirix P, Nuyts S, Van den Bogaert W. Radiation-induced xerostomia in patients with head and neck cancer: a literature review. *Cancer.* 2006 Dec 1; 107(11):2525-34.

[36] O'Sullivan EM, Higginson IJ. Clinical effectiveness and safety of acupuncture in the treatment of irradiation-induced xerostomia in patients with head and neck cancer: a systematic review. *Acupunct. Med.* 2010 Dec; 28(4):191-9.

[37] Wijers OB, Levendag PC, Braaksma MM, Boonzaaijer M, Visch LL, Schmitz PI. Patients with head and neck cancer cured by radiation therapy: a survey of the dry mouth syndrome in long-term survivors. *Head Neck.* 2002 Aug; 24(8):737-47.

[38] Cooperstein E, Gilbert J, Epstein JB, Dietrich MS, Bond SM, Ridner SH, et al. Vanderbilt Head and Neck Symptom Survey version 2.0: report of the development and initial testing of a subscale for assessment of oral health. *Head Neck.* 2012 Jun; 34(6):797-804.

[39] Coppes RP, Zeilstra LJ, Kampinga HH, Konings AW. Early to late sparing of radiation damage to the parotid gland by adrenergic and muscarinic receptor agonists. *Br. J. Cancer.* 2001 Sep 28; 85(7):1055-63.

[40] Shiboski CH, Hodgson TA, Ship JA, Schiodt M. Management of salivary hypofunction during and after radiotherapy. *Oral Surg. Oral Med. Oral Pathol. Oral Radiol. Endod.* 2007 Mar; 103 Suppl:S66 e1-19.

[41] Leek H, Albertsson M. Pilocarpine treatment of xerostomia in head and neck patients. *Micron.* 2002; 33(2):153-5.

[42] Epstein JB, Chin EA, Jacobson JJ, Rishiraj B, Le N. The relationships among fluoride, cariogenic oral flora, and salivary flow rate during radiation therapy. *Oral Surg. Oral Med. Oral Pathol. Oral Radiol. Endod.* 1998 Sep; 86(3):286-92.

[43] Chambers MS, Garden AS, Kies MS, Martin JW. Radiation-induced xerostomia in patients with head and neck cancer: pathogenesis, impact on quality of life, and management. *Head Neck.* 2004 Sep; 26(9):796-807.

[44] Epstein JB, Rea G, Wong FL, Spinelli J, Stevenson-Moore P. Osteonecrosis: study of the relationship of dental extractions in patients receiving radiotherapy. *Head Neck Surg.* 1987 Sep-Oct; 10(1):48-54.

[45] Epstein J, van der Meij E, McKenzie M, Wong F, Lepawsky M, Stevenson-Moore P. Postradiation osteonecrosis of the mandible: a long-term follow-up study. *Oral Surg. Oral Med. Oral Pathol. Oral Radiol. Endod.* 1997 Jun; 83(6):657-62.

[46] Hong CN, JJ; Hodgson BD, et al;. Dental Disease Section, Oral Care Study Group, Multi-national Association of Supportive Care in Cancer (MASCC)/International Society of Oral Oncology(ISOO). A systematic review of dental disease in patients undergoing cancer therapy. *Support Care Cancer.* 2010; 18:1007-21.

[47] de Graeff A, de Leeuw JR, Ros WJ, Hordijk GJ, Blijham GH, Winnubst JA. Long-term quality of life of patients with head and neck cancer. *Laryngoscope.* 2000 Jan; 110(1):98-106.

[48] Ruo Redda MG, Allis S. Radiotherapy-induced taste impairment. *Cancer Treat. Rev.* 2006 Nov; 32(7):541-7.

[49] Shi HB, Masuda M, Umezaki T, Kuratomi Y, Kumamoto Y, Yamamoto T, et al. Irradiation impairment of umami taste in patients with head and neck cancer. *Auris. Nasus. Larynx.* 2004 Dec; 31(4):401-6.

[50] Sandow PL, Hejrat-Yazdi M, Heft MW. Taste loss and recovery following radiation therapy. *J. Dent. Res.* 2006 Jul; 85(7):608-11.

[51] Lin A, Kim HM, Terrell JE, Dawson LA, Ship JA, Eisbruch A. Quality of life after parotid-sparing IMRT for head-and-neck cancer: a prospective longitudinal study. *Int. J. Radiat. Oncol. Biol. Phys.* 2003 Sep 1; 57(1):61-70.

[52] Oates JE, Clark JR, Read J, Reeves N, Gao K, Jackson M, et al. Prospective evaluation of quality of life and nutrition before and after treatment for nasopharyngeal carcinoma. *Arch. Otolaryngol. Head Neck Surg.* 2007 Jun; 133(6):533-40.

[53] Halyard MJ, A.; Sloan, JA; et al. . Does zinc sulfate prevent therapy-induced taste alterations in head and neck cancer patients? Results of phase III double-blind, placebo-controlled trial from the North Central Cancer Treatment Group (N01C4). *Int. J. Radiat. Oncol. Biol. Phys.* 2007; 67:1318-22.

[54] Nelson GM. Biology of taste buds and the clinical problem of taste loss. *Anat. Rec.* 1998 Jun; 253(3):70-8.

[55] McBride SM, Parambi RJ, Jang JW, Goldsmith T, Busse PM, Chan AW. Intensity-modulated versus conventional radiation therapy for oropharyngeal carcinoma: long-term dysphagia and tumor control outcomes. *Head Neck.* 2013 Apr; 36(4):492-8.

[56] Nangia S, Chufal KS, Tyagi A, Bhatnagar A, Mishra M, Ghosh D. Selective nodal irradiation for head and neck cancer using intensity-modulated radiotherapy: application of RTOG consensus guidelines in routine clinical practice. *Int. J. Radiat. Oncol. Biol. Phys.* Jan 1; 76(1): 146-53.

[57] Lambrecht M, Nevens D, Nuyts S. Intensity-modulated radiotherapy vs. parotid-sparing 3D conformal radiotherapy. Effect on outcome and toxicity in locally advanced head and neck cancer. *Strahlenther. Onkol.* Mar; 189(3):223-9.

[58] Tribius S, Bergelt C. Intensity-modulated radiotherapy versus conventional and 3D conformal radiotherapy in patients with head and neck cancer: is there a worthwhile quality of life gain? *Cancer Treat. Rev.* 2011 Nov; 37(7):511-9.

[59] Koukourakis MI, Danielidis V. Preventing radiation induced xerostomia. *Cancer Treat. Rev.* 2005 Nov; 31(7):546-54.

[60] Burlage FR, Roesink JM, Kampinga HH, Coppes RP, Terhaard C, Langendijk JA, et al. Protection of salivary function by concomitant pilocarpine during radiotherapy: a double-blind, randomized, placebo-controlled study. *Int. J. Radiat. Oncol. Biol. Phys.* 2008 Jan 1; 70(1):14-22.

[61] Berk L. Systemic pilocarpine for treatment of xerostomia. *Expert Opin. Drug Metab. Toxicol.* 2008 Oct; 4(10):1333-40.

[62] Lopez-Galindo MP, Bagan JV, Jimenez-Soriano Y, Alpiste F, Camps C. Clinical evaluation of dental and periodontal status in a group of oncological patients before chemotherapy. *Med. Oral Patol. Oral Cir. Bucal.* 2006 Jan; 11(1):E17-21.

[63] Chaveli López B, Gavaldá Esteve C, Sarrión Pérez MG. Dental treatment considerations in the chemotherapy patient. *J. Clin. Exp. Dent.* 2011; 3:e31-42.

[64] Wilberg P, Hjermstad MJ, Ottesen S, Herlofson BB. Chemotherapy-Associated Oral Sequelae in Patients With Cancers Outside the Head and Neck Region. *J. Pain Symptom Manage.* 2014 Apr 18.

[65] Nagler RM, Nagler A. Salivary gland involvement in graft-versus-host disease: the underlying mechanism and implicated treatment. *Isr. Med. Assoc. J.* 2004 Mar; 6(3):167-72.

[66] Imanguli MM, Alevizos I, Brown R, Pavletic SZ, Atkinson JC. Oral graft-versus-host disease. *Oral Dis.* 2008 Jul; 14(5):396-412.

[67] Jensen SB, Pedersen AM, Vissink A, Andersen E, Brown CG, Davies AN, et al. A systematic review of salivary gland hypofunction and xerostomia induced by cancer therapies: prevalence, severity and impact on quality of life. *Support Care Cancer.* 2010 Aug; 18(8):1039-60.

[68] Mosel DD, Bauer RL, Lynch DP, Hwang ST. Oral complications in the treatment of cancer patients. *Oral Dis.* 2011 Sep; 17(6):550-9.

[69] Dost F, Farah CS. Stimulating the discussion on saliva substitutes: a clinical perspective. *Aust. Dent. J.* 2013 Mar; 58(1):11-7.

[70] Hahnel S, Rosentritt M, Handel G, Burgers R. Influence of saliva substitute films on initial Streptococcus mutans adhesion to enamel and dental substrata. *J. Dent.* 2008 Dec; 36(12):977-83.

[71] Hahnel S, Behr M, Handel G, Burgers R. Saliva substitutes for the treatment of radiation-induced xerostomia--a review. *Support Care Cancer.* 2009 Nov; 17(11):1331-43.

[72] Jha N, Seikaly H, McGaw T, Coulter L. Submandibular salivary gland transfer prevents radiation-induced xerostomia. *Int. J. Radiat. Oncol. Biol Phys.* 2000 Jan 1; 46(1):7-11.

[73] Regelink G, Vissink A, Reintsema H, Nauta JM. Efficacy of a synthetic polymer saliva substitute in reducing oral complaints of patients suffering from irradiation-induced xerostomia. *Quintessence Int.* 1998 Jun; 29(6):383-8.

[74] Zhang Y, Guo CB, Zhang L, Wang Y, Peng X, Mao C, et al. Prevention of radiation-induced xerostomia by submandibular gland transfer. *Head Neck.* 2012 Jul; 34(7):937-42.

[75] Jha N, Harris J, Seikaly H, Jacobs JR, McEwan AJ, Robbins KT, et al. A phase II study of submandibular gland transfer prior to radiation for prevention of radiation-induced xerostomia in head-and-neck cancer (RTOG 0244). *Int. J. Radiat. Oncol. Biol. Phys.* 2012 Oct 1; 84(2):437-42.

[76] Blom M, Dawidson I, Fernberg JO, Johnson G, Angmar-Mansson B. Acupuncture treatment of patients with radiation-induced xerostomia. *Eur. J. Cancer B Oral Oncol.* 1996 May; 32B(3):182-90.

[77] Jedel E. Acupuncture in xerostomia--a systematic review. *J. Oral Rehabil.* 2005 Jun; 32(6):392-6.

[78] Braga FP, Lemos Junior CA, Alves FA, Migliari DA. Acupuncture for the prevention of radiation-induced xerostomia in patients with head and neck cancer. *Braz. Oral Res.* 2011 Mar-Apr; 25(2):180-5.

[79] Cowart BJ. Taste dysfunction: a practical guide for oral medicine. *Oral Dis.* 2011 Jan;17(1):2-6.

[80] Chaveli-Lopez B. Oral toxicity produced by chemotherapy: A systematic review. *J. Clin. Exp. Dent.* 2014 Feb; 6(1):e81-e90.

[81] Fark T, Hummel C, Hahner A, Nin T, Hummel T. Characteristics of taste disorders. *Eur. Arch. Otorhinolaryngol.* 2013 May; 270(6):1855-60.

[82] Boer CC, Correa ME, Miranda EC, de Souza CA. Taste disorders and oral evaluation in patients undergoing allogeneic hematopoietic SCT. *Bone Marrow Transplant.* 2010 Apr; 45(4):705-11.

[83] Yamashita H, Nakagawa K, Tago M, Nakamura N, Shiraishi K, Eda M, et al. Taste dysfunction in patients receiving radiotherapy. *Head Neck.* 2006 Jun; 28(6):508-16.

[84] Bergdahl M, Bergdahl J. Perceived taste disturbance in adults: prevalence and association with oral and psychological factors and medication. *Clin. Oral Investig.* 2002 Sep; 6(3):145-9.

[85] Caribe-Gomes F, Chimenos-Kustner E, Lopez-Lopez J, Finestres-Zubeldia F, Guix-Melcior B. Dental management of the complications of radio and chemotherapy in oral cancer. *Med. Oral.* 2003 May-Jul; 8(3):178-87.

In: Horizons in Cancer Research. Volume 55
Editor: Hiroto S. Watanabe
ISBN: 978-1-63463-228-7
© 2015 Nova Science Publishers, Inc.

Chapter 6

Psychoeducation: An Alternative for Preparing the Cancer Patient's Primary Caregiver

Vivian Guerra Morales[1]*, Lisandra Angulo Gallo[2]†,
Zeida Castillo Díaz[3]‡, Aguedo M. Treto González[4]§,
Maria Domingas Cassinda Vissupe[5]‖,
Mayté González García[6]♯, Rachel Fernández Ramos[7]**, Ladisbel
López Lorenzo[8]†† and Patricia Gil Pérez[9]‡‡

[1] Ph.D. in Psychological Sciences, Master in Health Psychology,
Central University "Marta Abreu" of Las Villas. Faculty of Psychology
[2] Psychology Graduate, Central University "Marta Abreu" of Las Villas,
Faculty of Psychology
[3] Ph.D. in Psychological Sciences, Master in Health Psychology,
Celestino Hernández Robau Oncology Hospital, Psycho-oncology Department
[4] MD. Specialist in Maxillofacial Surgery, Master in Health Psychology,
Celestino Hernández Robau Oncology Hospital
[5] Psychology Graduate, Master in Health Psychology, Pedagogic University of Bié,
[6] Psychology Graduate, University "Carlos Rafael Rodríguez" of Cienfuegos,
Faculty of Social Sciences and Humanities

* Email: viviang@uclv.edu.cu
† Email: lisandraa@uclv.cu
‡ Email: zeida@hchr.vcl.sld.cu
§ Email: treto@hchr.vcl.sld.cu
‖ Email: vissupe@yahoo.com.br
♯ Email: mgarciag@ucf.edu.cu
** Email: rachel.ffernandez@reduc.edu.cu
†† Email: ladisbel@fach.co.cu
‡‡ Email: patriciagp@hchr.vcl.sld.cu

[7] Psychology Graduate, University "Ignacio Agramonte Loynaz" of Camagüey,
Faculty of Psychology
[8] Psychology Graduate, University "José Martí" of Sancti Spíritus, Faculty of Humanities
[9] Psychology Graduate, Celestino Hernández Robau Oncology Hospital,
Psycho-oncology Department

Abstract

Introduction: Cancer is a chronic disease with a huge bio-psycho-social and spiritual impact not only for the patient but also for the caregiver, who generally does not have the preparation to deal with this difficult task.

Objective: To evaluate the effectiveness of the psychoeducational guides (PG) for the preparation of the primary caregiver of children and adults with cancer.

Methods and procedures: A pre-experimental, cross-sectional design, pre and post-test, was performed. The sample was selected intentionally and was formed by 95 caregivers, 42 children and 53 adults with oncological disease from different centers from the provinces of Havana, Villa Clara, Cienfuegos, Camaguey and Santiago de Cuba. For the study, methods such as observation, questionnaire and the psychological interview followed by a Likert scale were applied. For processing data, the Wilcoxon test, the qualitative analysis of verbalizations and the methodological triangulation were utilized.

Results: The results showed differences between the variables before and after the implementation of the PG. After the implementation of the PG results show positive influence in the knowledge of the disease, coping styles and motivation for the role ($p < 0.05$) of caregivers. There were no changes in the adoption of positive ways of life ($p = 0.655$, $p > 0.05$)

Conclusion: PG was effective in developing better care skills in primary caregivers of children and adults with cancer, regardless of their inclusion in psychosocial intervention programs.

Keywords: Psychoeducation, primary caregiver, cancer

1. Introduction

The human being is a bio-psycho-social and spiritual unity that works systemically thereby showing the relationship of the psyche and the body. The process of health-disease influences the lives of people. The impact of an oncological disease may be manifested in each patient and also in their family. (Garzón Pérez, 2013).

Cancer is currently a serious health problem in most of the countries. Statistics indicate that one in three people will develop the disease at some point in their life. This justifies the high rate of incidence, prevalence and mortality exhibited internationally and shows a trend to keep on rising day by day (World Health Organization, 2013).

In Cuba as in the majority of the countries, cancer is the leading cause of death (Ministry of Health, 2012). The gross rate of highest incidence occurred in men in the province of Villa Cara (537.5 x 100 000) prevailing lung cancer, skin cancer, prostate and colon cancer) as referenced in the National Cancer Registry (Ministry of Health, 2011). Moreover, there is a trend in women to be diagnosed with breast, skin, lung and cervical cancer. In the pediatric population diagnosis of leukemia, lymphoma, and tumors of the nervous system prevail.

Cancer has a huge psychological and social impact in population. Treatments used to control the disease are usually aggressive and affect the patients' physical and emotional status (Galindo, Álvarez-Avitia, Alvarado, 2013). The family of the patient also enter into crisis that sometimes overwhelms its adaptation possibilities, taking into account the adverse situation faced by assuming care responsibilities (Grau, Chacón, Reyes, 2012).

The unasked questions, the repressed feelings and the denied communication on issues related with the disease, are elements that are part of a phenomenon that some authors have called the silence conspiracy (Bermejo, Villacieros, Carabias Sánchez, Díaz-Albo, 2013). This issue together with the inability to provide proper and safe patient care, increased the caregiver's burden (Espín-Andrade, 2012).

Theses aspects point to the need to prioritize the comprehensive care of patients with cancer and also of their families, from inpatient and outpatient services, making them protagonists of the healing process (Cruzado, 2013)

To achieve this purpose Psychoeducation has become a valuable therapeutic tool, which encourage an institutional space that supports the patient and the caregiver from Health services (Johnson, 2003). It also encourages the active participation of the family from the start of treatment in collaboration with the healthcare team.

Since its origin, Psychoeducation was used as an interventional alternative for psychosocial rehabilitation of schizophrenic patients, with leading authors like Anderson, Reiss and Hogarty (1980, 1986, 1988). Now, it has been directed towards caregivers, in order to facilitate their understanding of the disease and provide support for living with a sick relative. There have been two major trends in the psychoeducational setting: one oriented to data transmission and the other oriented to propose behavioural changes in an intervention process (Colom, 2011)

Today it has emerged as a therapeutic modality in other diseases. Its application is encouraged, as Goldstein and Miklowitz (1995), in all family stress disorder which has a prognostic effect. It has proven effective in reducing relapses, high symptoms, family burden, emotional distress and concerns (Johnson, 2003; Soto-Pérez, 2011) in health issues such as bipolar disorder (Candini, Buizza, Girolamo, Ferrari, Caldera, Nobili, Pioli, Zanini, 2013; Candini, Buizza, Girolamo, Ferrari, Caldera, Nobili, Pioli, Zanini, 2013; Scott, Colom, Popova, 2009)), dementia (Espín-Andrade, 2009), depression (Casañas, Catalán, Raya, Real, 2014; Shimazu, Shimodera, Mino, Nishida, Kamimura Sawada, 2011), eating disorders (Geist, Heinmaa, Stephens, Davis, Katzman, 2000; Storch, Keller, Weber, Spindler, Milos, 2011), diabetes (Pibernik -Okanović , 2011), posttraumatic stress (Dorrepaal, Thomaes, Smit, Van Balkom, Veltman, Hoogendoorn, Draijer, 2012) and epilepsy (Rojas Sánchez, Alba Perez, Fardales Macías García, 2013)

Psychoeducation has been implemented in the area of psycho-oncology in both the caregivers and the patients with different types of cancer and locations, aimed at achieving better preparation of these people to adverse effects of medical treatment (Carmen, Richardson, Richardson, 2011; Jones, Cheng, Jackman, Walton, Haines, Rodin, Catton, 2013; Shimazu, Shimodera, Mino, Nishida, Kamimura, Sawada, 2011; Schou Bredal, Kåresen, Smeby, Espe, Sørensen, Amundsen, Aas, Ekeberg, 2014; Walker, 2013).

Psychoeducational guides (PG) are a form of Psychoeducation which has been implemented since 2009 by the authors of this chapter, as an alternative for helping cancer patients and their caregivers. Unlike brochures, manuals or other media the Psychoeducational guides are available for caregivers of cancer patients from various literature sources. They are based on a diagnosis of their needs and not only aimed at offering knowledge. Also, in a more personalized way and in line with the objectives and basic principles of Soto-Pérez (2012) seeks training caregivers to face their care deficiencies effectively, to develop skills and coping styles that allows them to live with the patient, reduce relapses and achieve the best social and occupational functioning.

The objective of this chapter is:

- To evaluate the effectiveness of psychoeducational guides for the preparation of primary caregiver of children and adults with cancer diseases, through its implementation.

2. Methods

The research was conducted from September 2012 to May 2013 in different health institutions in Cuba: "Celestino Hernández Robau" Oncology Hospital, "José Luis Miranda" Pediatric Hospital, Oncology and Radiobiology Institute (INOR), "Marie Curie" Oncology Hospital, "Héroes of Playa Girón" specialized Outpatient Center (CEA), and the "Conrado Benitez" Oncology Hospital. These constitute oncology centers of reference national and include psychology sevices. The directors of health institutes gave their consent for the study and agreed collaborate with the research process. A pre-experimental, cross-sectional study under a pre and post-test design was performed.

Operationalization of Variables

Independent Variable

Psychoeducation Guides: The design starts with a needs assessment of primary caregivers of children and adults with cancer, to guide them and prepare them for more efficient care. The guides used in the research are characterized by:

Description

These PG consist of four booklets aimed to prepare the caregiver regarding topics related with the care of children and adults with cancer. The central categories of each booklet are based on the essential psychoeducational needs of caregivers identified in studies (Alvarez & Sánchez, 2012; Roselló & Núñez, 2008). Each was developed separately, using a simple and easily understandable language for its users:

For Adults with Oncological Disease

- Learn more about how to be a good caregiver of adults with cancer.
- Do you know how to provide emotional support to the person you care about?
- Do you know about the nutritional necessity of a cancer patient?
- How to control the side effects of chemotherapy?

For Children with Oncological Disease
- What is cancer?
- General characteristics of treatment in children with oncological disease.
- Care of the child with oncological disease.
- How to manage my emotions.

The guides were evaluated strictly by specialists and users and were refined to achieve the final version of the guides (García-Soto, 2012; Treto, 2009). The contribution of experienced professionals in different topics such as psychologists, oncologists, radiotherapists, chemotherapists, nutritionists, paediatricians, nurses, journalists, statisticians was essential to achieve this purpose.

Dependent Variable
Operational definition of the Preparation of primary caregiver: Process that enables the acquisition of information about the disease, treatment, adequate nutrition, emotional support to the patient, control of emotions of the caregiver and the child care, enhancing effective coping styles in primary caregiver and stimulating the motivation for the role and skills in the caregiver.

- Knowledge of the disease: Includes providing information of the characteristics of oncological diseases and its treatment (definition, etiology, manifestations, classification, nutrition, treatment and prognosis).
- Coping styles: Efforts needed to deal with the demands that go beyond the primary caregiver, regardless of their effectiveness or their intrinsic value (acceptance, positive reinterpretation, positive life changes and confrontation, role of caregiver, seeking important information, seeking social support).
- Motivation for the role: Combination of physiological, psychological and social processes on the suffering family member or friend that forces a person to act with energy in the care process. It is related to the attachment that connects the patient with the caregiver.

(These indicators were subjected to an evaluation of 16 specialists linked to the health care of patients, which expressed their agreement with the operational definition diseases offered).

Intervening Variables
Commitment to care: Commitment of primary caregiver to spend time, energy and effort to the attention of the sick person.

Experience as a primary caregiver: Previous experiences related to care of someone.

The PG is considered effective if they increase awareness of the disease, stimulate the development of effective coping styles and encourage motivation for caregiver role.

Participants

The sample was formed by 95 primary caregivers of relatives with cancer, selected from an intentional sampling. The participant should meet the following criteria: be the primary caregiver of a patient diagnosed with cancer, the patients with a diagnostic phase of the disease (children) or clinical stage III and IV receiving chemotherapy (adults), provide consent to participate and cooperate in the research and to belong to health institutions referred to in the context of research. Participants showed to have different educational levels, rural and urban origins, of both sexes, with various cancer diagnoses.

Procedures

In order to investigate the psycho-educational needs and coping styles of the main caregivers during the support and care of children and adults with cancer a semi structured interview accompanied by a Likert scale (ranging from 1 to 5, where 1 means no preparation, 2 poor preparation, 3 medium preparation, 4 sufficient preparation and 5 optimal preparation) was used and participant observation. These techniques were repeated after the application of the Psychoeducational guides.

Data were processed using the statistical package SPSS for Windows, version 18.0. Descriptive statistics were used in addition to the Wilcoxon test before and after the implementation of the PG. In addition, a qualitative analysis of the information like verbalizations emitted by the subject was used for methodological triangulation.

3. Results

The particpants were 95 caregivers of cancer patients, belonging to both child and adolescent stage (42) to adult (53) from the provinces of Havana, Cienfuegos, Villa Clara, Camaguey and Santiago de Cuba. In relation to their sociodemographic characteristics, it was evident a predominance of females (92.6%) and age ranges between 31-50 years (57.9%).

It was also found that most of them are from urban areas (74.7%), with different levels of education, prioritizing the 12th grade (48.4%) and equivalence in the presence or absence of employment (47.4%) respectively.

Carers of children were all mothers 95, 5 % (40), in the case of the adult were children (34 %), and brothers (20, 8 %).

Regarding the diagnosis, most types of neoplasms in children were leukemia (38,1 %) and lymphomas (28,6 %), and breast cancer (15.8%) and lung cancer (28,3%) in adults (17,2 %). In children the evolution time of the disease was less than a month. Adults had an evolution time of 1 to 5 years since the diagnosis.

After reading the PG, all the participants showed satisfaction with its design ensuring that images, colours and text promote the right understanding of each booklet. They also referred to language as understandable and clear with the size and font used, a fact that encourages a greater understanding of the psychoeducational resource. They also expressed the need to have them all the time, proposing alternatives for its access.

Figure 1 show the results emerged from comparing preparation of caregivers, pre and post reading the Psychoeducational guide, taking into account specifically the knowledge about the oncological disease.

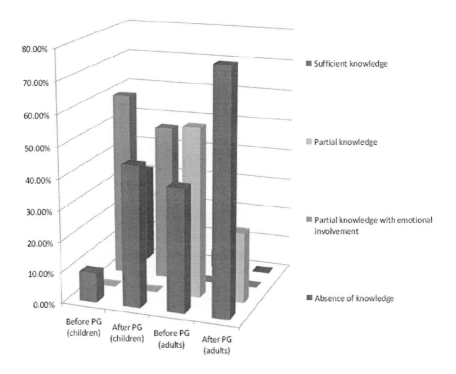

Figure 1. Knowledge of the disease in caregivers of cancer patients, before and after the implementation of the PG.

In general, Wilcoxon test revealed significant differences among the caregivers. (p=0.00; p>0.05).

The first interview showed that caregivers of children with cancer have partial knowledge of the disease, affective involvement in 59.5% (25) ("The most terrible thing I know, leads to death"), which remained in 21 of these in the second evaluation and noting an increased by 28.3% (15) of those with adequate knowledge.

Caregivers of adults 21 (39.6%) seemed to express a wide knowledge of the disease, prognosis, treatment, nutrition, etc. increasing this number after reading the PG (77.4%). An interesting finding is that there is an unequal distribution among caregivers of children and caregivers of adults, possible explained from the time that caregivers of adults exercise this role, which is lower in the case of the caregivers of children. Another indicator that came out in the study is that the participants improve their care skills after the reading of the PG. ("Now I know how to move forward, communicate and listen to my relative, I can be a better support right now").

Similarly, there were found changes related to coping styles at the health situation, in favor of increased adaptive styles, which is illustrated in Table 1.

Table 1. Comparison between coping styles of caregivers, before and after the implementation of the PG

Indicators	Wilcoxon test sig.	Compariso n	Sig.	Decision
Disease Acceptance	0.000	<	0.05	Reject the invalid hypothesis
Positive reinterpretation	0.025	<	0.05	Reject the invalid hypothesis
Positive Lifestyle changes	0.655	>	0.05	Accept the invalid hypothesis
Confrontation	0.000	<	0.05	Reject the invalid hypothesis
Acceptance of caregiver's role	0.000	<	0.05	Reject the invalid hypothesis
Seek of useful information	0.000	<	0.05	Reject the invalid hypothesis
Seek of social support	0.000	<	0.05	Reject the invalid hypothesis

It was evident, as a generality, a considerable rise mainly to search for information (children: 47, 6% strongly agree increased to 73.8%, adults: 71% increased to 81%).

Similarly, caregivers of adults with cancer increase the seeking of social support from 52.8% to 73.6%. In addition, from 15 (28.3%) who didn't assume confrontational behaviors, only two remained in this position.

The main changes in caregivers of children were related to the motivation for the role (from 69% to 90.5%). These were also highlighted by the lack of support as a search strategy. Only 5 (11.9%) had this strategy before reading the PG, and 7 (16.7%) eventually recognized the need to seek help from others.

Changes didn't occur in the adoption of positive life changes where scores remained virtually unchanged. The 73.8% (31) and 28.3% (15) of caregivers of children and adults, respectively, was not in accordance with the sentence: "I have made positive changes in my life to cope with the disease of my relative", yielding lower percentages in the caregivers of children.

The PG also influenced the motivation of caregivers to perform the work. Significant differences were found in relation to this indicator, in both times of assessment ($p = 0.00$, $p > 0.05$). The results are displayed in Figure 2, showing a significant increase in favour of the adoption of an intrinsic motivation, based on the bond with the family.

In adult caregivers the changes were more discrete, because the first evaluation, 92.5% (49) showed no motivation for this work.

Only 2 of the 59.5% caregivers of children who had negative results in this area, kept this condition ("I still cannot get used to it, but I still have to assume it"). As mentioned above, these caregivers had little time in their role, which justify they show more resistance to changes in lifestyle such as assuming this role.

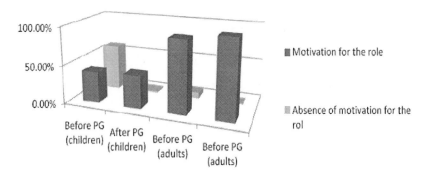

Figure 2. Motivation for the role in caregivers of cancer patients, before and after the implementation of the PG.

4. Discussion

The sociodemographic characteristics of participants are quite similar to those of other studies (Carrillo, Barrera, Sanchez, Carrreño, Chaparro, 2014; Montero, Jurado, Méndez, 2014), which shows that the person responsible for exercising the role of caregiver (specially caregiver of children) is usually female, middle aged, mostly the mother. This is influenced by existing gender stereotypes.

It was significant the prevalence of a partial knowledge of the disease with emotional involvement in caregivers of children. The knowledge was negatively influenced by social taboos and representations in relation to cancer. These conceptions of the disease should not be dismissed, because they are a representation of the meaning of cancer by the patient and family and it is important to diagnose their attitude towards the disease. We agree with Builes & Bedoya (2006), by stating that the disease has three levels of meaning: biological, symbolic and social dimension. Psychoeducation should work from these dimensions to promote the construction of new meanings that favor the intervention process.

Although the PG managed changes in caregivers offering a more complete view of the oncological disease, they should be considered as an auxiliary tool of systematic work and comprehensive psychoeducational care provided to patients and their families. Longitudinal studies developed by Walker (2013), showed that the Psychoeducational Guide was helpful to increase awareness of the side effects of treatment and how to deal with them, but the study didn't demonstrate a decrease of the side effects and relieve of emotional distress after the application.

The PG also succeeded in respect of improving the coping styles in caregivers. However they didn't significantly influence the lifestyles of caregivers and the adoption of healthy habits to achieve higher psychosocial wellbeing. According to the authors this could be a dimension, difficult to change because these are stable and rooted personality patterns. However, PG were affective in improving the seeking of information and a better understanding, especially in caregivers for children, who showed significant differences I the pre and post evaluation. Similar results related to coping styles was found and founded by Espada and Grau (2012) referring the tendency to isolation and lack of seeking social support.

Changes in motivation for the role of caregivers were also seen in both groups, however those caregivers of children stand out. It is believed that the knowledge and skills to care acquired, plus the emotional support offered by the PG, facilitated this outcome, however this incentive should be systematically encouraged.

Conclusion

The PG proved to be effective to have a positive impact on the preparation of the primary caregiver of children and adults with cancer disease, regardless of their empowerment to include them in psychoeducational programs. They helped to increase knowledge about the disease; they favoured the adoption of effective coping styles, encouraged motivation for the role in caregivers, and finally developed care skills in participants. This last variable was incorporated into the operational definition of preparation of the primary caregiver of children with cancer. The psychoeducational guides should be consider useful as part of a comprehensive, multidisciplinary approach to treatment of oncologic disease.

References

[1]   Alvarez, Y., Sánchez, D. (2012). *Guía Psicoeducativa para familiares de niños (as) con enfermedad oncológica.* (trabajo de diploma no publicado) Universidad Central "Marta Abreu" de Las Villas, Santa Clara.

[2]   Anderson, C. M., Reiss, D. J., y Hogarty, G. E. (1988). *Esquizofrenia y familia: guía práctica de psicoeducacion.* Buenos Aires: Amorrortu.

[3]   Bermejo, J.C., Villacieros, M., Carabias, R., Sánchez, E., Díaz-Albo, B. (2013). Conspiración del silencio en familiares y pacientes al final de la vida ingresados en una unidad de cuidados paliativos: nivel de información y actitudes observadas. *Medicina Paliativa,* 20 (2), 49–59. doi: 10.1016/j.medipa.2012.07.002

[4]   Builes, M.V., Bedoya, M.H. (2006). La psicoeducación como experiencia narrativa: comprensiones posmodernas en el abordaje de la enfermedad mental. *Revista Colombiana de Psiquiatría*, 35 (4), 463-475.

[5]   Candini, V., Buizza, C., Girolamo, G., Ferrari, C., Caldera, M.T., Nobili, G.,... Pioli, R., Zanini, A. (2013). Astudy of effectiveness of structured group psychoeducation for bipolar patients. A controlled trial in Italy *European Psychiatry 28*(1), 1-12. doi: org/10.1016/S0924-9338(13)76164-9

[6]   Carmen, W.H., Richardson, A., Richardson, J. (2011). Managing Symptoms in patients with Advanced Lung Cancer During Radiotherapy: Results of a Psychoeducational Randomized Controlled Trial. *Journal of Pain and Symptom Management, 41*(2), 347–357. Recuperado de: http://dx.doi.org/10.1016/j.jpainsymman.2010.04.024

[7]   Casañas, R., Catalán, R., Raya, A., Real, J. (2014). Efectividad de un programa grupal psicoeducativo para la depresión mayor en atención primaria: ensayo clínico controlado aleatorizado. *Revista de la Asociación Española de Neuropsiquiatría, 34*(121), 145-146. doi: 10.4321/S0211-57352014000100009

[8]   Carrillo, G.M., Barrera, L., Sánchez, B., Carrreño, S.P., Chaparro, L. (2014). Efecto del programa de habilidad de cuidados para cuidadores familiares de niños con cáncer. Revista Colombiana de Cancerología, 18 (1),18-26.

[9]   Colom, F. (2011). Psicoeducación, el litio de las psicoterapias. Algunas consideraciones sobre su eficacia y su implementación en la práctica diaria. *Revista Colombiana de Psiquiatría, 40*, 147-165.

[10]   Cruzado, J.A. (2013) . *Manual de psicooncologia: Tratamientos psicológicos en pacientes con cáncer.* (pp. 79-100). Madrid: Pirámide.

[11]   Dorrepaal, E., Thomaes, K., Smit, J.H., Van Balkom, A.J., Veltman,D.J., Hoogendoorn, A.W., Draijer, N. (2012). Stabilizing Group Treatment for Complex Posttraumatic Stress Disorder Related to Child Abuse Based on Psychoeducation and Cognitive Behavioural Therapy: A Multisite Randomized Controlled Trial. *Psychother Psychosom* (81), 217–225. doi: 10.1159/000335044

[12]   Espada, M.C. y Grau, C. (2012). Estrategias de afrontamiento en padres de niños con cáncer. *Psicooncología, 9,* (1), 25-40.

[13]   Espín Andrade, A. M. (2009). "Escuela de Cuidadores" como programa psicoeducativo para cuidadores informales de adultos mayores con demencia. *Revista Cubana de Salud Pública*, 35, 0-0. Recuperado de: http://scielo.sld.cu/scielo.php?script=sci_arttext&pid= S0864-3466200 9000200019&nrm=iso

[14]   Espín Andrade, A. M. (2012). Factores de riesgo de carga en cuidadores informales de adultos mayores con demencia. *Revista Cubana de Salud Pública,* 38, 493-402. Recuperado de: http://scielo.sld.cu/scielo.php?script=sci_arttext&pid=S0864-3466201 2000300006&nrm=iso

[15]   Galindo, O., Álvarez Avitia, M., Alvarado, S. (2013). Ansiedad, depresión y afrontamiento en pacientes con cáncer testicular en tratamiento y periodo de seguimiento. *Psicooncología,* 10(1), 69-78. doi:10.5209/rev_PSIC.2013.v10.41948

[16]   García-Soto, N. (2012). *Evaluación de una Guía Psicoeducativa para cuidadores principales de niños con enfermedades oncológicas.* (trabajo de diploma no publicado) Universidad Central "Marta Abreu" de Las Villas, Santa Clara.

[17]   Garzón Pérez, A. (2013). Transformaciones y nuevas perspectivas profesionales y académicas de la Psicología de la Salud. *Revista Latinoamericana De Psicologia, 45*(2), 241-252. doi:http://dx.doi.org/10.14349/rlp.v45i2.596

[18]   Geist, R., Heinmaa, M., Stephens, D., Davis, R., Katzman, D.K. (2000). Comparison of family therapy and family group psychoeducation in adolescents with anorexia nervosa. *Canadian Journal of Psychiatry. Revue Canadienne de Psychiatrie 45*(2), 173-178.

[19]   Goldstein, M. J., y Miklowitz, D. J. (1995). The effectiveness of psychoeducational family therapy in the treatment of schizophrenic disorders. *Journal of Marital and Family Therapy, 21*(4), 361-376.

[20]   Grau, J., Chacón, M., Reyes, M. (2012); *Guías de cuidados para familiares de enfermos crónicos avanzados.* La Habana: Editorial Ciencias Médicas.

[21]   Jones, J.M., Cheng, T., Jackman, M., Walton, T., Haines, S., Rodin, G., Catton, P. (2013). Getting back on track: evaluation of a brief group psychoeducation intervention for women completing primary treatment for breast cancer. *Psycho-Oncology, 22* (1), 117–124. doi: 10.1002/pon.2060

[22]   Johnson, D. L. (2003). *Family Education or Behavioral Family Psychoeducation: Making a Choice.* Ponencia presentada en el Segundo Encuentro de Organizaciones Familiares de Latino América, World fellowship for schizophrenia and allied disorder (WFSAD).

[23] Medina, Y. (2010). *Evaluación de la calidad de la Guía Psicoeducativa para el cuidador principal de pacientes oncológicos en estadío III y VI, en tratamiento quimioterapéutico.* (trabajo de diploma no publicado), Universidad Central "Marta Abreu" de Las Villas, Santa Clara.

[24] Ministerio de Salud Pública. (2012). Anuario Estadístico de Salud. La Habana: Dirección Nacional de Estadísticas. Disponible en: http://bvscuba.sld.cu/blog /2013/04/29/anuario-estadistico-de-salud-2012/

[25] Ministerio de Salud Pública. (2011). Registro Nacional de Cáncer. Disponible en: http:// www. Uncc.sld.cu/

[26] Montero, X., Jurado, S., Méndez, J. (2014). Carga, ansiedad y depresión en cuidadores primarios informales de niños con cáncer. *Psicología de la Salud*, 24 (1), 45-53.

[27] Roselló, D.M., Núñez, Y. (2008). Elaboración de una *Guía Psicoeducativa para el cuidador principal del paciente con enfermedad oncológica en estadio clínico III y IV con tratamiento quimioterapéutico.* (trabajo de diploma no publicado) Universidad Central "Marta Abreu" de Las Villas, Santa Clara.

[28] Organización Mundial de la Salud (OMS). (2013). *Estadísticas sanitarias mundiales.* Disponible en: www.who.int

[29] Pibernik-Okanović. (2011). Does treatment of subsyndromal depression improve depression and diabetes related outcomes: protocol for a randomised controlled comparison of psycho-education, physical exercise and treatment as usual. *Trials,* 12, 17. Recuperado de: http://www.trialsjournal.com/content/12/1/17

[30] Rojas, G.A., Alba, L., Fardales, V.E., García, J. (2013). Intervención psicoeducativa dirigida a personas con epilepsia y sus familiares. *Gaceta Médica Espirituana, 15*, 272-283.

[31] Schou Bredal, I., Kåresen, R., Smeby, N.A., Espe, R., Sørensen, E.M., Amundsen, M., Aas, H., Ekeberg, Ø. (2014).Effects of a Psychoeducational Versus a Support Group Intervention in Patients With Early-Stage Breast Cancer: Results of a Randomized Controlled Trial. *Cancer Nursing, Publish Ahead of Print*,37(3) doi: 10.1097/NCC.0b013e31829879a3

[32] Scott, J., Colom, F., Popova, E. (2009). Long-term mental health resource utilization and cost of care following group psychoeducation or unstructured group support for bipolar disorders: a cost-benefit analysis. *The Journal of Clinical Psychiatry,* 70, 378-86.

[33] Shimazu, K., Shimodera, S., Mino, Y., Nishida, A., Kamimura, N., Sawada, E. (2011). Family psychoeducation for major depression: randomised controlled trial. *The British Journal of Psychiatry*, 338–340. doi: 10.1192/bjp.bp.110.078626

[34] Soto-Pérez, F., De vena-Diez, V., Lucas-Cardoso, E., Bueno-Aguado, Y., Orihuela-Villamerriel, T., y Franco-Martín, M. (2011). Ciberterapias: el uso de internet en Salud Mental: Experiencias en el mundo y posibilidades en Chile. En *Socializar Conocimientos* (pp. 259-264). Barcelona: Icaria.

[35] Soto-Pérez, F., Franco-Martín, M., Losada, R., Rodríguez, C., Cid, T., y Hornero, R. (2011). Psychoed: Online Alternatives for Caregiver's Support of Handicapped People. En M. Jordanova y F. Lievens (Eds.), *Online Global Telemedicine and e Health Updates, Knowledge Resources* (Vol. 4, pp. 238-241). Luxemburgo: Medetel.

[36] Storch, M., Keller, F., Weber, J., Spindler, A., Milos, G. (2011). Psychoeducation in Affect Regulation for Patients with Eating Disorders: A Randomized Controlled Feasibility Study. *American Journal of Psychotherapy, 65*(1), 81-93.

[37] Treto, A. (2009). *Validación de una Guía Psicoeducativa para el cuidador principal del paciente con enfermedad oncológica en estadio clínico III y IV con tratamiento quimioterapéutico.* (tesis de maestría no publicada). ISCM. "Serafín Ruíz de Zárate Ruíz", Santa Clara.

[38] Walker, L. M. (2013). *A Psycho-Education Intervention to Help Men with Prostate Cancer Adapt to Androgen Deprivation Therapy.* (Disertación doctoral no publicada) Universidad de Calgary, Alberta.

Index

#

20th century, 45, 79

A

access, 128, 140
accounting, 49
acetylcholine, 109, 110
acid, 3, 34, 74, 75, 79, 83, 84, 87, 88, 89, 97, 98, 100, 110, 120
acidic, 21, 109, 113, 115, 121, 124
acne, 5
acupuncture, ix, 101, 109, 111, 112, 113, 120, 121, 128, 131
acute promyelocytic leukemia, viii, 71, 72
adaptation, 137
adenine, 79, 80
adenocarcinoma, 12, 14, 17, 20, 22, 28, 33, 40, 91
adenoma, 47, 50, 54, 58, 66, 78
adhesion, 26, 53, 85, 133
adolescents, 145
ADP, 3, 74
adults, x, 44, 53, 134, 136, 138, 140, 141, 142, 144
adverse effects, 28, 84, 86, 89, 110, 137
AFM, 2, 14
agar, 7
age, 31, 44, 45, 54, 103, 106, 130, 140
aggressiveness, 54, 58, 65
agonist, 88, 109, 110
AIDS, 125
albumin, 124, 127
algorithm, 57, 58, 59, 60, 62, 66
alkaloids, 6
allele, 56, 68
allergic reaction, 108
alpha-tocopherol, 108

alters, 40
amino, 4, 9, 51, 74, 80
amino acid(s), 4, 9, 51
amino groups, 74
ammonia, 124
amphibia, 89
amylase, 105, 124
amyloidosis, ix, 123, 125
anabolism, 16
analgesic, 104
anatomy, 103
anchorage, 24
androgen, 80, 91, 98
angiogenesis, 15, 16, 30, 34, 40, 80, 82, 83, 93
angiotensin converting enzyme, 16
angle closure glaucoma, 109
anorexia, 5, 145
anorexia nervosa, 145
antiangiogenic, vii, 1
antibody, 84
anti-cancer, 21
anticancer activity, 7, 8, 9, 21, 32
anticancer drug, 10, 96
antidepressants, 104
antidiabetic, vii, 1
antigen, 15, 115
antihistamines, 104
anti-inflammatory, vii, 1, 5, 12, 31, 84
antimicrobial, vii, 1, 125, 129
antioxidant, vii, 1, 5, 12, 24, 74
antitumor, 8, 18, 80, 84, 98
antitumor agent, 8
antitumorigenic effect, vii, 1
antiviral, vii, 1
anxiety, 106, 125
APC, 55
APL, viii, 71, 72, 80, 85, 86, 89
apnea, 106

apoptosis, viii, 3, 9, 10, 11, 12, 13, 14, 15, 17, 18, 19, 20, 22, 23, 24, 25, 26, 27, 28, 29, 30, 32, 33, 34, 35, 36, 37, 38, 39, 40, 41, 42, 47, 52, 53, 71, 74, 76, 77, 80, 82, 83, 84, 85, 88, 93, 94, 95, 96, 97, 98, 99, 100, 126, 130
apoptosis pathways, 34
appetite, 104, 112
Argentina, 72
arrest, viii, 14, 28, 29, 41, 71, 83, 86, 98, 99
arsenic, vii, ix, 72, 73, 74, 79, 80, 84, 85, 86, 89, 90, 91, 92, 93, 94, 95, 96, 97, 98, 99
arsenic poisoning, 73
arsenic trioxide, vii, 72, 73, 79, 90, 91, 92, 93, 94, 95, 96, 97, 98, 99
arteriosclerosis, 72
arthritis, 36, 103
aryl hydrocarbon receptor, 15, 34
ascites, 15, 34
ascorbic acid, 81, 83, 92, 96
aspiration, vii, 43, 45, 62, 63, 64, 68, 69
assessment, 38, 56, 68, 88, 131, 138, 142
asthenia, 109
asthma, 5, 79, 109
atherosclerosis, 5, 15
ATO, viii, ix, 71, 72, 79, 80, 81, 82, 83, 84, 85, 86, 88, 89, 92
ATP, 19, 73
atrophy, 105, 113
attachment, 26, 139
Austria, 71, 73
autoimmune disease(s), ix, 54, 103, 117, 123, 125
autoimmune disorders, ix, 101, 102, 103
autoimmunity, 115
autonomic nervous system, ix, 123
autophagy, viii, 21, 36, 71, 79, 82, 83, 85, 88, 91, 95, 98
autosomal dominant, 47, 54
awareness, 102, 139, 143

B

bacteria, ix, 123, 125, 126
behaviors, 44, 45, 142
benefits, 4, 90, 107, 108, 112
benign, 45, 46, 47, 48, 49, 50, 51, 53, 58, 59, 66, 69
Bethesda system, vii, 43, 46
beverages, 109
bicarbonate, 125
bile, 110
bioavailability, 17, 21, 28
biological activities, 32
bioluminescence, 16
biomarkers, 46, 52, 69

biopsy, 45, 62, 63
biosynthesis, 32, 33
bipolar disorder, 137, 146
black tea, 5, 16
bladder cancer, 82, 83, 94
bleeding, 102
blood, 14, 15, 60, 64, 68, 88, 105, 111, 121
blood flow, 111
blood supply, 15
blood vessels, 88, 105
bloodstream, 25, 26, 49
bone, 85, 98, 115, 127
bone marrow, 127
brain, 88
Brazil, 123
breakdown, 21, 115, 126
breast cancer, 4, 23, 24, 25, 26, 27, 38, 39, 40, 80, 81, 82, 83, 84, 85, 92, 93, 95, 96, 97, 140, 145
breast carcinoma, 81, 83
breathing, 103, 106
bronchospasm, 109
brothers, 140
buccal mucosa, 111, 124

C

Ca^{2+}, 18, 20, 22, 37, 96
CAF, 2, 24
caffeine, 105, 115
calcitonin, 54, 112, 120
calcium, 103, 111, 125, 126, 128
CAM, 31
cancer cells, 8, 11, 12, 13, 14, 15, 17, 18, 19, 21, 22, 24, 25, 26, 27, 35, 37, 40, 41, 69, 80, 83, 84, 91, 94, 95, 96, 97, 104
cancer death, 17, 44, 45
cancer stem cells, 21, 83, 97
cancer therapy, 126, 127, 129, 131
candidiasis, 102, 106, 115, 128
carcinogen, 16, 19, 72
carcinogenesis, 8, 12, 13, 18, 33, 40, 83
carcinogenicity, viii, 71, 72
carcinoma, 9, 12, 13, 16, 18, 19, 26, 29, 33, 35, 37, 39, 40, 41, 44, 45, 46, 50, 52, 53, 54, 56, 58, 60, 61, 62, 63, 64, 65, 66, 67, 68, 78, 80, 81, 82, 83, 84, 85, 87, 88, 89, 90, 92, 93, 94, 95, 96, 97, 98, 99, 100, 132
caregivers, x, 136, 137, 138, 140, 141, 142, 143, 144
caries, 115, 125, 129
cascades, 76, 77, 94
Caspase-8, 14
caspases, 13
categorization, 6, 49

category a, 57

Caucasians, 47

CD26, 91

CDK inhibitor, 13

cDNA, 114

cell culture, 17, 96

cell cycle, viii, 13, 15, 24, 41, 71, 76, 83, 86, 93, 95

cell death, 9, 14, 18, 19, 20, 21, 25, 27, 28, 31, 35, 40, 66, 88, 91, 93, 94, 96, 97, 99, 100

cell differentiation, 51, 94

cell division, 53

cell invasion, viii, 26, 30, 39, 72, 77, 90

cell invasiveness, 94, 95

cell line(s), ix, 9, 12, 13, 14, 15, 16, 17, 18, 19, 20, 21, 22, 23, 24, 25, 26, 27, 28, 35, 37, 38, 39, 40, 41, 48, 72, 80, 82, 83, 84, 85, 88, 89, 93, 94, 97, 98, 99, 100

cell movement, 13

cellular energy, 21

cellular growth factors, 47

central nervous system (CNS), ix, 41, 92, 123

cervical cancer, 41, 81, 84, 91, 93, 95, 98, 137

cervix, 80, 82, 83, 84, 85

challenges, viii, 43

cheilitis, 115

chemical, 6, 128

chemoprevention, 30

chemopreventive agent(s), vii, 1, 5, 19, 33, 36

chemoradiation, ix, 101, 117, 130

chemosensitizer, vii, 1, 11, 19, 42

chemotherapeutic agent, 8, 9, 22

chemotherapeutic compound, viii, 71

chemotherapy, viii, ix, 11, 13, 18, 19, 22, 24, 37, 70, 71, 83, 87, 97, 103, 105, 118, 123, 124, 125, 126, 127, 128, 129, 130, 132, 133, 134, 138, 140

Chicago, 91

childhood, 81, 92, 129

childhood cancer, 129

children, x, 44, 49, 64, 73, 136, 138, 139, 140, 141, 142, 143, 144

Chile, 72, 146

China, 72, 80

Chinese medicine, 79, 94, 111

cholangiocarcinoma, 83, 95

choline, 110

chromosome, 22, 23, 75

chymotrypsin, 20

cigarette smoke, 12, 33

cigarette smoking, 115

City, 43

civilization, 4

clarity, vii, 43

classes, 4, 104, 105

classification, 45, 46, 59, 63, 65, 68, 69, 139

cleavage, 14, 18

clinical application, 56, 69

clinical diagnosis, 57

clinical trials, vii, viii, ix, 2, 28, 30, 31, 48, 61, 71, 72, 80, 81, 87, 88, 89, 102, 111, 116

clusters, 106

CMC, 110

codon, 84, 97

coffee, 5

colic, 5

collaboration, 137

collagen, 113

collateral, 127

colon, vii, 1, 19, 20, 21, 22, 35, 36, 37, 78, 80, 82, 84, 85, 94, 97, 99, 136

colon cancer, 20, 21, 22, 36, 37, 80, 82, 84, 85, 94, 97, 99, 136

color, vii, 1, 5, 6

colorectal adenocarcinoma, 21, 22

colorectal cancer, viii, 16, 20, 22, 23, 34, 36, 37, 38, 48, 71, 83, 97

combination therapy, 97

commercial, vii, 2, 28, 57

communication, vii, 43, 137

complement, 46, 57

compliance, 38

complications, 86, 114, 117, 118, 126, 127, 129, 130, 133, 134

composition, 6, 103, 105, 106, 111, 115, 127, 129

compounds, vii, viii, ix, 1, 4, 6, 19, 23, 32, 72, 73, 74, 79, 80, 85, 88, 90, 124, 126

computed tomography, 45

conference, 46, 62

confrontation, 139

Congress, 37, 69

conjugation, 74

connective tissue, ix, 103, 106, 118, 124, 125, 126

consensus, 46, 103, 121, 129, 132

consent, 138, 140

conspiracy, 137

constipation, 5

constituents, 5

construction, 143

consumption, 109, 115

control group, 12, 19, 24

controlled trials, 112, 115

controversial, 49

cooking, 5

coordination, 56

COPD, 109

copper, 24

correlation, 21, 27, 33, 64, 85, 100, 127

cost, 57, 60, 107, 108, 112, 146
cost-benefit analysis, 146
cough, 5
creatinine, 124
cross-sectional study, 138
CSCs, 25, 26
CT, ix, 16, 20, 124, 126, 127, 128
Cuba, x, 136, 138, 140
culture, 15, 22, 96
culture medium, 15
Curcuma longa, vii, 1, 5, 6, 31, 32, 33
curcumin, vii, 1, 2, 6, 7, 8, 9, 10, 12, 13, 15, 18, 21, 22, 23, 24, 25, 27, 28, 30, 31, 32, 33, 34, 35, 36, 37, 38, 39, 40, 41, 42
cure, 4, 7, 108
cyclins, 60
cyclooxygenase, 23
cyclophosphamide, 18, 104, 105
cystatins, 124
cysteine, 74
cystic fibrosis, ix, 103, 123, 125
cytochrome, 80
cytokines, 26, 39, 77
cytologic examination, 48
cytologic samples, viii, 44, 49, 58, 59, 60, 61
cytology, vii, 43, 44, 57, 58, 60, 61, 68, 69
cytometry, 18
cytoplasm, 20, 21, 86
cytoprotectant(s), ix, 101, 107
cytoskeleton, 13, 14, 36, 88, 94
cytostatic drugs, ix, 72
cytotoxic agents, 9
cytotoxicity, 12, 18, 22, 24, 28, 73, 79, 96, 107

D

database, 57
deacetylation, 87
deaths, 8, 13, 25
decay, ix, 102, 114, 123, 125
defects, 13, 22
deficiency(s), 15, 50, 53, 138
degradation, 11, 15, 21, 84, 86
dehydration, 103, 106
dementia, 137
dental caries, 126, 128, 129
dentures, 115, 125
dephosphorylation, 21
depolarization, 80
deposits, 72
depression, 106, 125, 137, 146
deregulation, 51
derivatives, 86

dermatology, 130
destruction, 14, 105, 106
detection, 11, 44, 45, 49, 51, 52, 56, 57, 58, 63, 64, 68, 69
detoxification, 74
diabetes, 5, 72, 103, 106, 125, 137, 146
diagnostic markers, 52
diarrhea, 5, 28, 72
diet, 12, 127
differential diagnosis, 60
diffusion, 128
dimensionality, 68, 69
dimerization, 10, 54, 76
direct action, 127
directors, 138
discharges, 5
discomfort, 110, 114, 125
diseases, vii, ix, 1, 4, 5, 7, 8, 28, 32, 47, 79, 101, 102, 103, 106, 125, 137, 138, 139
disorder, ix, 101, 103, 106, 111, 137, 145
distilled water, 111
distribution, 34, 49, 80, 90, 105, 107, 127, 141
diversity, 6
dizziness, 109
DNA, viii, 13, 21, 22, 24, 25, 27, 36, 37, 40, 51, 54, 56, 65, 72, 79, 82, 86, 87, 94, 95, 99, 107, 126
DNA damage, 24, 79, 126
DNA sequencing, 54
docetaxel, 89
DOI, 34, 62
donors, 127
dosage, 73
dosing, 108
double blind study, 116
down-regulation, 11, 12, 15, 16, 19, 20, 22, 25, 26, 27, 29, 30, 33, 34, 38, 39, 41, 67, 83, 95, 96
DPO, 57
drinking water, 72
drug delivery, 93
drug discovery, vii, 2
drug efflux, 19, 35
drug resistance, 11, 22
drug synergy, vii, 2, 18
drug testing, 61
drugs, vii, viii, ix, 2, 9, 11, 16, 19, 23, 27, 32, 46, 71, 83, 84, 85, 87, 88, 89, 94, 95, 97, 103, 104, 110, 118, 123, 125, 127, 128
dry eyes, 111
dry mouth, ix, 101, 102, 103, 104, 105, 109, 111, 112, 113, 115, 116, 118, 119, 120, 123, 125, 130, 131
drying, 115
dyspepsia, 5

dysphagia, 132

E

eating disorders, 137
E-cadherin, 16, 30, 34, 41
ecology, 129
ecosystem, 124
eczema, 79
editors, 63, 65, 67, 117
education, 58, 140, 146
elders, 118
electron, 21
electron microscopy, 21
electrophoresis, 14
e-mail, 1
emboli, 93
embolization, 93
emotional distress, 137, 143
employment, 140
empowerment, 144
enamel, 125, 133
encephalitis, ix, 123, 125
encoding, 121
endocrine, 44, 45, 47, 54, 67, 73, 78, 83, 89, 96
endocrine system, 78
endometrial carcinoma, 94
endothelial cells, 14, 15, 16, 80, 85
energy, 139
environment(s), 15, 103
enzyme(s), 2, 13, 20, 30, 60, 73, 74, 110
epigenetic alterations, 21
epilepsy, 137
epithelial cells, 9, 12, 27, 33, 39, 44, 106, 128
epithelium, ix, 44, 53, 64, 123, 126
erythrocytes, 73
erythropoietin, 15
ESO, 28
esophageal cancer, vii, 1, 40
esophagus, 128
estrogen, 24, 38, 83, 96
ethnic background, 106
etiology, 118, 129, 130, 139
eukaryotic, 76
evidence, ix, 31, 47, 53, 59, 63, 65, 101, 102, 108, 112, 113, 128
evolution, 56, 69, 140
excision, 13, 112
exercise, 141
exons, 54
expenditures, 57
expertise, 113

exposure, ix, 9, 18, 47, 49, 50, 53, 72, 73, 86, 91, 101, 107
extracts, 110
extrusion, 73
EZH2, 3, 24, 38

F

families, 47, 137, 143
family history, 21
family members, 10, 23, 47, 51, 54, 60, 79
family therapy, 145
FAS, 3, 14, 16
fat, 16, 20
fatty acids, 15, 16
FDA approval, 10
fear, 106, 125
feelings, 137
fibroblasts, 2, 10, 24, 38, 73, 83, 86
fibrosarcoma, 85
fibrosis, 5, 36, 105
fibrous cap, 51
films, 107, 133
financial, 57
fish, 47
fixation, 56
flatulence, 5, 110
flavor, vii, 1, 5, 128
flora, 110, 126, 131
fluid, 99, 103, 104, 114, 127, 128
fluorescence, 51, 56
FNA, vii, 43, 44, 45, 46, 47, 48, 55, 59, 60, 61, 69
folate, 73, 80
folklore, vii, 1
follicular lesion, vii, 43, 44, 46, 51, 58, 60, 61, 68
food, vii, 1, 4, 5, 12, 128
food additive, 5
Food and Drug Administration (FDA), 3, 5, 10, 56, 61, 87, 108, 109
force, 2
formation, vii, 1, 14, 18, 20, 22, 26, 37, 74, 80, 87, 113, 125, 129
formula, 6
France, 34
free radicals, 12, 107
fruits, 5
functional changes, 126
fungal infection, 115
fusion, 49, 51, 64, 65

G

gallbladder, 40, 95
gastrointestinal tract, 23
gel, 115, 128
gene amplification, 12, 78
gene expression, 12, 17, 25, 27, 37, 49, 51, 58, 60, 63, 65, 66, 69, 96
gene regulation, 89
gene transfer, ix, 101, 114, 121
genes, viii, 9, 13, 14, 15, 17, 20, 21, 25, 30, 32, 33, 44, 47, 48, 49, 50, 51, 52, 53, 56, 57, 59, 74, 86, 87, 95
genetic abnormalities, viii, 43
genetic alteration, 54, 66
genetic defect, 20
genetic marker, 57
genetic mutations, 67
genetics, 64, 90
genome, 93
genomic instability, 21
genomics, 95, 99
genotyping, 65
genus, 6
germ cells, 41
Germany, 71
ginger, vii, 1, 5
gingival, 128
gingivitis, 102, 114
gland, ix, 101, 102, 103, 104, 105, 107, 108, 109, 111, 114, 115, 119, 121, 123, 124, 125, 126, 127, 128, 132, 133
glioblastoma, 82, 84, 96, 97, 98
glioblastoma multiforme, 97
glioma, viii, 41, 71, 80, 81, 82, 83, 84, 85, 96, 98
glucose, 34, 82, 89, 124
glutathione, 12, 33, 73, 74, 84, 88, 91, 94, 99
glycolysis, 73
goiter, 44, 47, 50, 55, 73, 89
granules, 109
granulomas, 106
GRAS, 5
growth, 3, 4, 9, 12, 13, 15, 18, 20, 22, 24, 25, 26, 27, 29, 30, 33, 35, 36, 37, 38, 40, 41, 51, 52, 60, 61, 69, 73, 74, 76, 77, 79, 80, 83, 89, 91, 93, 95, 96, 115, 125, 126, 127
growth arrest, 36, 80
growth factor, 3, 4, 24, 25, 30, 37, 38, 52, 60, 61, 69, 76, 77, 79, 95, 125, 126, 127
guidelines, 88, 109, 111, 112, 117, 118, 132

H

half-life, 17
halitosis, 102, 125
HCC, 13
head and neck cancer, ix, 81, 92, 101, 102, 103, 117, 118, 119, 120, 121, 129, 130, 131, 132, 133
head and neck radiotherapy, ix, 124, 126
headache, 28
healing, 125, 137
health, 4, 8, 17, 31, 103, 124, 129, 136, 137, 138, 139, 140, 141
health care, 8, 139
health care system, 8
heart disease, 109
hematuria, 5
hemochromatosis, ix, 123, 125
hemorrhage, 6
hepatitis, 106
hepatocellular carcinoma, viii, 13, 16, 33, 34, 35, 71, 81, 83, 85, 92, 94, 96, 97, 98
hepatocytes, 73, 82, 90, 94
hepatoma, 15, 34, 80, 82, 83, 84, 85, 93, 97, 99
hepatotoxicity, 73
heterogeneity, 44, 49, 56, 64
histidine, 74
histology, 47, 50, 55, 88
histone, viii, 19, 21, 36, 72, 79, 82, 83, 84, 87, 128
histone deacetylase, viii, 72, 82, 83, 84, 87, 128
history, 5, 53, 109
HM, 91, 93, 118, 119, 132
homeostasis, 90, 124
homocysteine, 73, 74
homogeneity, 107
hormone(s), 20, 73, 77, 89
hormone levels, 73
hormone-refractory prostate cancer, viii, 71, 80, 92
host, 15, 106, 114, 124, 127, 132
HPV, 41
hTERT, 60
human, 4, 5, 7, 9, 11, 12, 13, 14, 15, 16, 17, 18, 19, 20, 22, 23, 24, 25, 26, 27, 28, 29, 30, 31, 32, 33, 34, 35, 36, 37, 38, 39, 40, 41, 42, 64, 66, 72, 78, 90, 91, 93, 94, 95, 96, 97, 98, 99, 100, 114, 116, 121, 129, 130, 136
hybridization, 56
hydro–electrolytic balance, ix, 123
hydrogen, 12
hydrogen peroxide, 12
hydroxyl, 12, 20
hydroxypropyl cellulose, 111
hygiene, 114, 126, 128
hyperactivity, 115

hyperbaric oxygen therapy, ix, 101, 109, 121
hypermethylation, 79, 91
hyperparathyroidism, 54
hyperplasia, 54
hypertension, 72
hyperthermia, 81, 83, 85, 92, 93, 99
hypotension, 108
hypothesis, 142
hypothireoidism, ix, 123, 125
hypothyroidism, 54, 73
hypoxia, 15, 34
hypoxia-inducible factor, 34

I

ID, 35, 38, 39, 63
ideal, 12, 59
identification, 36, 48, 62
idiopathic, 36, 114
IL-8, 3, 12, 17, 20
images, 140
imaging modalities, 45
immunofluorescence, 26
immunoglobulin(s), 105, 124, 127
immunohistochemistry, 57, 60, 68
immunostimulatory, 84
improvements, 112, 115
in situ hybridization, 51
in vitro, vii, 1, 7, 9, 12, 14, 15, 16, 17, 20, 21, 24, 25,
    26, 28, 30, 31, 34, 35, 36, 39, 40, 41, 56, 80, 89,
    91, 93, 94, 95, 96, 97, 99, 100
in vivo, vii, 1, 13, 14, 21, 25, 26, 28, 30, 36, 39, 80,
    91, 93, 94, 95, 96, 99
incidence, 8, 23, 44, 45, 47, 49, 52, 72, 78, 84, 86,
    103, 105, 126, 136
income, 8
index case, 60
India, vii, 1, 5, 28, 31, 72
individuality, 46
individuals, 44, 47, 53, 103
indolent, 45, 54
induction, viii, 10, 13, 20, 21, 30, 33, 38, 39, 40, 41,
    71, 80, 82, 83, 85, 91, 93, 94, 95, 96, 98, 99
infection, 102, 128
inflammation, 5, 26, 28, 77, 102
inflammatory disease, 106
ingestion, 20
ingredients, 6
inheritance, 47, 54
inhibition, 12, 13, 14, 15, 16, 18, 20, 21, 22, 23, 25,
    26, 29, 30, 33, 34, 37, 38, 39, 41, 74, 75, 76, 80,
    82, 83, 84, 87, 91, 93, 94, 95, 97, 98, 115

inhibitor, 2, 3, 12, 15, 16, 18, 19, 23, 26, 27, 29, 39,
    40, 41, 48, 83, 84, 86, 87, 93
initiation, 19, 21, 76, 90
injections, 79
injury, 5, 105
inositol, 75, 78
institutions, 60, 138, 140
insulin, 52, 60, 126
integrin, 26, 29, 39
integrity, 125, 128
interference, 4
interferon, 34, 97
interleukin-8, 33, 36
interphase, 56, 57
intervention, x, 54, 136, 137, 143, 145
intestine, 28
intracellular calcium, 96
intrinsic motivation, 142
intrinsic value, 139
introns, 50
involution, 109
iodine, vii, 47, 49, 50, 53, 58, 73, 87, 90, 99, 100,
    124
ionizing radiation, ix, 47, 50, 72, 83, 84, 85
ions, 124
iritis, 109
iron, ix, 72, 85
irradiation, ix, 23, 98, 105, 107, 109, 119, 121, 124,
    131, 132, 133
irrigation, 124
irritable bowel syndrome, 5
ischemia, 72
Islam, 92
isolation, 6, 143
issues, 17, 112, 137
Italy, 31, 144

J

jaundice, 5
joint destruction, 36
journalists, 139

K

K^+, 124
Kaposi sarcoma, 10
keratoconjunctivitis, 106
kidney, viii, 71, 72, 81
kinase activity, 29

L

Lactobacillus, 126
lactoferrin, 124
laryngeal cancer, 95
larynx, 94, 95, 124, 128
lead, 21, 78, 102, 106, 109, 128
legend, vii, 1
lesions, viii, 19, 36, 43, 44, 45, 46, 49, 51, 53, 56, 57, 59, 60, 61, 68, 69, 72, 88, 92
leucine, 77
leukemia, 3, 35, 42, 79, 80, 92, 99, 137, 140
life changes, 139, 142
ligand, 2, 14, 29, 41, 48, 60
light, 3
Likert scale, x, 136, 140
liposomes, 80, 93
liver, vii, 1, 3, 9, 13, 14, 15, 16, 17, 34, 72, 85, 90, 93, 94, 99
liver cancer, 13, 14, 15, 16, 17, 34, 99
liver disease, 3, 16
liver metastases, 16, 34
liver transplant, 13
liver transplantation, 13
lobectomy, 59
localization, 67
loci, 47, 56
locus, 77
longitudinal study, 132
low risk, 112
lubricants, 111, 115, 116
lung cancer, viii, 3, 4, 9, 11, 12, 13, 33, 71, 81, 82, 83, 84, 85, 90, 96, 97, 98, 136, 140
lung metastases, 88
Luo, 37, 97, 98
lupus, 5
lymph, 47, 48, 49, 88
lymph node, 47, 48, 49, 88
lymphocytes, 106
lymphoma, 2, 10, 54, 137
lysozyme, 124

M

magnesium, 111, 127
magnetic resonance, 45
magnetic resonance imaging, 45
major depression, 146
majority, 20, 25, 44, 46, 47, 52, 54, 102, 136
malignancy, viii, 44, 45, 46, 51, 53, 57, 58, 59, 60, 61, 78, 118
malignant tumors, 127

management, vii, ix, 43, 45, 48, 53, 56, 58, 59, 61, 63, 66, 68, 101, 108, 117, 118, 119, 120, 126, 127, 129, 130, 131, 134
mandible, 113, 131
manipulation, 112
Marx, 100
mass, 14, 18, 69, 87
mass spectrometry, 18
matrix, 14, 30, 34, 41
matrix metalloproteinase, 14, 30, 34, 41
matter, 6
MB, 23, 24, 25, 26, 27, 38, 39, 40, 62, 120
measurement(s), 112, 114, 130
mechanical stress, 77
media, 138
median, 45, 64
medical, 4, 79, 90, 103, 137
medication, viii, 71, 85, 102, 103, 104, 110, 134
medicine, vii, 1, 4, 5, 8, 31, 32, 79, 111, 133
medulla, 54
MEK, 30, 42, 51, 77, 78
melanoma, viii, 10, 48, 71, 80, 81, 82, 83, 92, 94
melt, 56
membranes, 107
mental health, 146
mesentery, 15
mesothelioma, 82, 93
meta-analysis, 109, 117
metabolic syndrome, 16
metabolism, ix, 13, 15, 66, 72, 73, 74, 82, 89
metabolites, 17, 28, 74
metal ion(s), 77
metalloproteinase, 3, 84
metamorphosis, 89
metastasis, 12, 13, 15, 16, 25, 26, 30, 33, 39, 41, 44, 47, 49, 91
metastatic disease, 47, 48, 52, 88
metformin, 83, 96
Methamphetamine, 104
methyl group(s), 19, 74
methylation, 21, 36, 79, 87
Mexico, 72
mice, 12, 13, 15, 16, 18, 20, 26, 34, 40, 83, 85, 93, 95, 98
microRNA, 50
microscope, 18
microscopy, 2
migration, viii, 13, 14, 16, 20, 21, 22, 24, 26, 33, 34, 36, 39, 51, 71, 77, 83, 85, 94, 98
mimicry, 4, 14, 34
miniature, 114
mitochondria, 4, 10, 22, 29, 52, 79, 80, 94
mitochondrial DNA, 52

mitochondrial pathway, viii, 32, 71, 82, 94, 97
mitogen, 29, 37, 41, 47, 67, 77, 96, 97
MMA, 74
MMP, 3, 13, 16, 26, 27, 29, 30, 33, 38, 39, 40
MMP-2, 13, 27, 29, 40
MMP-9, 13, 16, 26, 29, 33
models, vii, viii, 1, 12, 21, 71, 72, 80, 85, 87, 130
modifications, 21, 128
moisture, 112
molecular marker, vii, 43, 46, 53, 56, 59, 61, 66, 67, 69
molecular medicine, vii
molecules, vii, 2, 10, 74, 105
monoclonal antibody, 60, 115
Moon, 39, 99
morbidity, 21, 102
morphogenesis, 77
morphology, 114
mortality, vii, 1, 9, 10, 11, 16, 19, 23, 25, 44, 136
mortality rate, 44
motif, 2, 50
motivation, x, 136, 139, 142, 143, 144
MR, 118
mRNA, 3, 4, 12, 14, 17, 22, 25, 26, 29, 60, 76, 95
mucin, 103, 126
mucosa, 23, 110, 115, 125, 127, 128
mucous membrane(s), 124
multiple factors, 8
multiple myeloma, 30, 41
muscarinic receptor, 109, 131
mutagen, 19
mutant, 12, 22, 48, 97
mutation(s), viii, 4, 44, 48, 49, 51, 52, 53, 54, 55, 56, 57, 58, 59, 60, 61, 62, 63, 64, 65, 66, 67, 68, 69, 78, 79, 84, 87, 90, 91
myelosuppression, 127
myofibroblasts, 24

N

Na$^+$, 68, 124
nanoparticles, 80, 93
narcotic, 4
nasopharyngeal carcinoma, 40, 80, 93, 98, 119, 132
nausea, 108, 109, 112
neck cancer, 120, 132, 133
necrosis, 4, 29, 88, 100, 105, 115, 126
negative effects, 124
neoplasm, 46, 47, 59, 78
neovascularization, 16, 77, 113
nephritis, 5
nerve, 113, 120, 121, 128
nerve fibers, 113, 128

nervous system, 10, 137
neuroblastoma, 91, 96
neurons, 111
neuroprotective agents, 5
neurosurgery, ix, 123, 125
next generation, 58
NH$_2$, 74, 77, 97
nitric oxide, 74
nitric oxide synthase, 74
nitrogen, 124
NMR, 32
nodules, vii, 43, 45, 46, 47, 48, 49, 50, 56, 58, 59, 60, 62, 63, 64, 68, 69
non-avid thyroid cancer, vii
normal aging, 102
NPC, 28, 40
Nrf2, 74, 82, 94
nuclei, 57
nucleic acid, 19
nucleotide sequencing, 68
nucleus, 20, 86
nurses, 139
nutraceutical, 4, 8
nutrients, 79
nutrition, ix, 4, 101, 102, 117, 132, 139, 141
nutritional deficiencies, 102

O

obesity, 26
obstruction, 106
oesophageal, 40
OH, 62, 69, 100
oil, 6
Oklahoma, 43
oleic acid, 16, 35
oncogenes, 30, 78
oncogenesis, 51
oncoproteins, 49
opportunities, 24
optimization, 48, 127
oral cavity, 10, 102, 105, 115, 124, 128, 130
oral health, ix, 101, 123, 124, 127, 129, 131
oral health problems, 127
organ(s), vii, 2, 25, 28, 30, 42, 57, 118
outpatient, 137
ovarian cancer, 82, 84, 85, 96
oxidation, 15, 16, 38, 72, 79
oxidative damage, 24
oxidative stress, 14, 25, 74, 79, 96, 97
oxide nanoparticles, ix, 72, 85
oxygen, 4, 12, 15, 74, 85, 90, 98, 113
oxygen consumption, 85, 98

oxygen consumption rate, 98

P

p16INK4A, 24
p53, viii, 9, 13, 21, 22, 25, 26, 27, 29, 30, 37, 38, 41, 52, 53, 57, 66, 67, 68, 72, 76, 84, 97, 126
paclitaxel, 27, 40, 83, 84, 97
pain, 5, 72, 81, 103, 104, 111, 112, 113, 116
palate, 124
palliative, 87, 89
palpation, 46, 63
pancreas, 82, 91
pancreatic cancer, 40, 80, 82, 83, 96, 97
paracentric inversion, 48, 49
parasympathetic nervous system, 110, 111, 113
parathyroid, 54
parenchyma, 105, 106
parotid, 102, 105, 107, 109, 118, 119, 124, 125, 126, 131, 132
parotid gland, 102, 105, 107, 118, 126, 131
participant observation, 140
participants, 88, 140, 141, 143, 144
patents, 8
pathogenesis, 61, 65, 78, 120, 131
pathologist, 47, 51
pathology, 56, 61
pathophysiology, 38
pathways, 10, 20, 23, 30, 32, 34, 51, 52, 54, 57, 61, 65, 76, 77, 78, 82, 84, 85, 87, 97, 115
patient care, 137
PCR, 4, 17, 25, 26, 56, 57, 60, 68
PCT, 68
pedigree, 47
penetrance, 47, 54
peptidase, 91
peptide, 18, 112, 120
perchlorate, 73, 89
perineum, 5
periodontal, ix, 123, 125, 126, 132
periodontal disease, ix, 123, 125, 126
peripheral blood, 48
peripheral nervous system, 111
permeability, 79
peroxide, 12
personality, 143
pesticide, 72
pH, 77, 105, 115, 124, 125
pharmaceutical, 4, 80
pharmacokinetics, 28
pharmacological agents, ix, 101, 108, 113
pharmacological effects, vii, 1
pharmacological treatment, 113

pharmacotherapy, 130
pharynx, 10, 40, 124
phenolic compounds, 6
phenotype(s), 21, 24, 27, 49, 51, 67
pheochromocytoma, 54
phosphate, 73, 75, 88, 111, 125, 126, 127
phosphatidylserine, 18
phosphorylation, 13, 16, 18, 22, 23, 24, 25, 27, 29, 30, 35, 39, 41, 76, 86, 91, 97
physical exercise, 146
PI3K, viii, 25, 27, 29, 30, 34, 39, 41, 51, 55, 72, 75, 76, 78, 79, 82, 85, 98
PI3K/AKT, 27, 34, 39, 55
pigs, 114
pilot study, 23, 38, 92, 121
placebo, 99, 109, 110, 112, 115, 116, 132
plants, 4, 6
plaque, 126
plasma levels, 72
plasma membrane, 21, 75, 105
plasminogen, 26, 39
PM, 97, 118, 132
point mutation, 48, 54, 56, 65, 68
poison, 4, 72
policy, 31
polymer, 84, 133
polymerase, 3, 4, 17, 20, 74
polymerase chain reaction, 4, 17
polymerization, 80, 99
polymorphism, 56
polypeptide, 3, 78, 112, 120
polyphenols, 5
polysaccharide(s), 96, 110
population, 32, 47, 58, 68, 107, 130, 137
posttraumatic stress, 137
potassium, 79, 111, 128
preparation, x, 104, 136, 137, 138, 140, 141, 144
preservation, 56, 107, 108
preservative, 5
prevention, ix, 4, 23, 25, 101, 102, 108, 109, 112, 117, 118, 119, 127, 129, 133
primary caregiver(s), vii, x, 136, 138, 139, 140, 144
primary cirrhoses, ix, 123, 125
primary tumor, 25, 88
priming, 57
principles, 138
probability, 61
proband, 54
probe, 57
professionals, 102, 139
profit, 60, 87, 88
progenitor cells, 105
progesterone, 24, 38

prognosis, ix, 13, 24, 44, 46, 47, 48, 51, 56, 60, 67, 72, 78, 87, 139, 141
proliferation, 12, 13, 14, 15, 16, 17, 18, 20, 21, 22, 23, 24, 25, 26, 27, 28, 29, 30, 34, 38, 39, 40, 41, 45, 47, 51, 54, 76, 79, 80, 82, 84, 86, 88, 91, 95
proline, 124
promoter, 48, 50, 51, 76, 83, 86, 91
prophylactic, 54, 118
prostate cancer, viii, 26, 41, 71, 80, 82, 83, 85, 91, 92, 98
prostate carcinoma, 81
proteasome, 20, 36, 86, 88
protection, 4, 73, 107, 124
protein analysis, 18
protein kinase C, 20
protein kinases, 30, 37, 76, 97
protein synthesis, 76
proteins, viii, 4, 15, 18, 19, 20, 21, 24, 28, 29, 51, 71, 74, 75, 124, 125
proteome, 14, 34
proteomics, 95
proto-oncogene, 66, 67, 75
psoriasis, 79
psychoeducational guides, x, 136, 138, 144
psychoeducational program, 144
psychology, 138
PTEN, 52, 53, 55, 60, 66, 75, 79
pyrimidine, 18

Q

quality of life, ix, 101, 102, 103, 117, 120, 121, 123, 125, 126, 127, 129, 130, 131, 132, 133
questionnaire, x, 114, 116, 130, 136

R

radiation, ix, 22, 23, 48, 49, 53, 64, 81, 83, 85, 87, 88, 89, 91, 92, 98, 100, 101, 102, 103, 105, 106, 107, 108, 109, 110, 112, 113, 114, 116, 117, 118, 119, 120, 121, 124, 127, 129, 130, 131, 132, 133
radiation damage, 131
radiation therapy, 22, 92, 100, 102, 103, 105, 107, 119, 124, 131, 132
radiation treatment, 88, 89, 98
radicals, 12, 80
radio, viii, 22, 48, 58, 61, 72, 78, 86, 87, 88, 90, 99, 100, 118, 134
radiosensitization, 30
radiosensitizer, vii, 1, 22, 42

radiotherapy, ix, 22, 98, 105, 107, 108, 111, 113, 114, 116, 117, 118, 119, 120, 121, 123, 124, 125, 126, 128, 129, 130, 131, 132, 133
reactions, 75, 76, 83
reactive oxygen, 85, 99, 126
reading, 140, 141, 142
real time, 17
receptors, 29, 48, 61, 77, 95, 110, 113, 127, 128
recognition, 47, 129, 130
recombination, 64
recommendations, 46, 113, 121
recovery, 103, 105, 107, 131
recruiting, 88
recurrence, 45, 47, 48, 68
recycling, 73
red wine, 5
regeneration, 105, 111
Registry, 136
rehabilitation, 137
relapses, 22, 137, 138
relatives, 140
relevance, 62, 66
relief, 110, 112, 115, 121, 128, 129
remission, 78
renal cell carcinoma, 41, 91
repair, 3, 22
replication, 15
repression, 18, 22, 26, 96
residues, 74, 75
resistance, 3, 8, 11, 12, 19, 22, 23, 24, 33, 35, 48, 83, 142
resolution, 56
resource utilization, 146
respiration, 85
response, 3, 21, 22, 33, 34, 58, 74, 81, 91, 103, 113
responsiveness, 61
resveratrol, 33, 37
reticulum, 3, 15, 35
retinoblastoma, 82, 83, 94, 95
reverse transcriptase, 60
rhinitis, 109
ribose, 3, 74
risk(s), 19, 26, 36, 46, 47, 48, 54, 57, 58, 59, 60, 61, 67, 68, 100, 107, 108, 114, 115, 118, 125, 126, 129
RNA(s), 3, 4, 17, 20, 56, 60, 76, 84
RNAi, 4, 21
roots, 5
rosiglitazone, 88, 100
Royal Society, 35

S

safety, 99, 110, 131
SAHA, 87
saliva, ix, 102, 103, 105, 107, 108, 109, 110, 111, 112, 113, 116, 118, 120, 121, 123, 124, 125, 126, 127, 128, 129, 130, 133
salivary flow, ix, 103, 105, 106, 107, 109, 110, 111, 112, 113, 114, 115, 116, 123, 125, 126, 127, 131
salivary gland(s), ix, 102, 103, 104, 105, 106, 107, 110, 111, 112, 113, 114, 115, 116, 117, 118, 119, 121, 123, 124, 125, 126, 127, 128, 130, 133
salivary substitutes, ix, 101, 109, 111, 116, 120
salts, 91
sarcoidosis, ix, 106, 123, 125
SAS, 28
savings, 57
scavengers, 14
schizophrenia, 145
schizophrenic patients, 137
science, 62
scripts, 31
SCT, 133
secretagogues, ix, 101
secretion, 20, 79, 103, 110, 112, 113, 124, 128, 129
sedatives, 104
sediments, 72
selectivity, 93, 119
senescence, 21, 24, 36, 38, 88
sensation, ix, 113, 123, 125
sensitivity, viii, 19, 52, 56, 57, 59, 60, 61, 72, 85, 91, 98, 109
sensitization, 11, 83
sequencing, 56, 58, 69
serine, 3, 26, 75, 76
serotonin, 23, 37
serum, 60, 124
services, 137
SES, 129
sex, 130
sham, 121
shock, 72
showing, 136, 142
sialic acid, 124
siblings, 127
side effects, ix, 27, 40, 85, 102, 108, 109, 110, 123, 126, 138, 143
signal transduction, 25, 77, 103, 105
signaling pathway, 13, 14, 16, 22, 23, 24, 25, 26, 27, 28, 30, 33, 34, 37, 39, 41, 42, 74, 78, 94, 98, 104
signalling, viii, 47, 48, 51, 53, 54, 63, 72, 87
signals, 14, 57, 76, 90
signs, 54

sinusitis, 5
siRNA, 4, 12, 14, 18, 21, 26, 36
skin, 10, 72, 92, 102, 112, 136
skin cancer, 10, 136
sleep disturbance, 102, 117
smooth muscle, 24
snacking, 106
social support, 139, 142, 143
sodium, 19, 35, 48, 51, 87, 90, 103, 111, 127, 128
software, 18
solid carcinomas, viii, 71, 80, 81
solid tumors, 15, 16, 45, 79, 98, 99, 127
solution, 6, 32, 79, 111, 116
somatic alterations, 51
somatic cell, 60
somatic mutations, 47, 51, 59
Spain, 37
specialists, 139
species, 4, 74, 85, 90, 99, 126
speech, ix, 101, 108, 114, 117, 124
sprain, 5
squamous cell, 40, 94
squamous cell carcinoma, 40, 94
SS, 92, 97, 106, 108, 110, 114, 118
stability, 15, 29, 41
standardization, 58
starvation, 21
state(s), 9, 21, 62, 63, 72, 102, 107
statin, 88
statistics, 7, 8, 58, 130, 140
stem cell replacement, ix, 101, 114
stem cells, 21, 36, 83, 91, 96, 105, 113, 114, 116
stereotypes, 143
sterols, 6
stimulant, 73, 104
stimulation, 76, 78, 89, 103, 111, 112, 113, 120, 121, 125, 128
stimulus, 77
stomach, vii, 1, 9, 17, 18, 35
stratification, 61
stress, 18, 21, 35, 74, 77, 85, 89, 125, 137
stress response, 74
stroma, 119
structure, 6, 32
Styria, 73
subgroups, 44, 65
submandibular gland, ix, 101, 102, 105, 108, 119, 121, 128, 133
substitutes, ix, 101, 109, 111, 116, 120, 128, 133
substitution(s), 4, 51
substrate, 4, 21, 36, 77
suicide, 18
sulfur, 74

Sun, 33, 38, 41, 93, 94, 96

supplementation, 108

suppression, viii, 15, 16, 25, 26, 30, 33, 39, 41, 71, 97, 127, 130

surgical intervention, viii, 43

surgical removal, 58, 106

surgical resection, 86

survival, 9, 12, 13, 16, 20, 21, 22, 23, 24, 30, 33, 36, 42, 44, 45, 47, 48, 51, 54, 61, 76, 78, 82, 83, 87, 96, 126

survival rate, 12, 24, 44, 45, 78

survivors, 126, 129, 131

susceptibility, 47

Switzerland, 31

symptoms, 54, 102, 103, 104, 105, 107, 108, 109, 111, 113, 115, 116, 117, 121, 125, 126, 127, 130, 137

syndrome, 47, 50, 106, 115, 116, 118, 121, 130, 131

synergistic effect, 11, 12, 16, 18, 84, 96

synthesis, 6, 16, 42, 76, 94, 99

syphilis, 79

T

T cell, 111

tamoxifen, 83

target, viii, 12, 13, 15, 20, 24, 25, 28, 35, 43, 67, 72, 74, 76, 79, 83, 86, 88, 89, 96, 99

techniques, 49, 56, 107, 140

technological advances, 63

teeth, 110, 115

teratogen, 19

testing, 56, 57, 59, 60, 61, 62, 63, 64, 68, 80, 93, 131

testing program, 93

TGF, 4, 13, 27, 39, 52, 77

therapeutic effects, viii, ix, 71, 72

therapeutic efficacy, viii, 71, 92, 98

therapeutic interventions, ix, 72

therapeutic targets, 14

therapeutic use, vii, 1

therapy, viii, ix, 10, 11, 14, 16, 18, 38, 46, 48, 58, 61, 62, 68, 72, 78, 83, 86, 87, 88, 89, 90, 92, 96, 100, 101, 103, 105, 114, 127, 128, 132

thickening agents, 110

threonine, 3, 4, 20, 75, 76

threshold level, 103

thyroglobulin, 51, 86, 100

thyroid, vii, viii, ix, 30, 41, 43, 44, 45, 46, 47, 48, 49, 50, 51, 52, 53, 54, 55, 56, 57, 58, 59, 60, 61, 62, 63, 64, 65, 66, 67, 68, 69, 70, 71, 72, 73, 78, 80, 83, 87, 88, 89, 90, 91, 95, 99, 100, 103, 106

thyroid cancer, vii, viii, ix, 30, 41, 44, 45, 46, 47, 48, 50, 53, 54, 56, 57, 60, 61, 62, 63, 64, 65, 66, 67,

68, 69, 70, 71, 72, 78, 83, 87, 88, 89, 90, 91, 95, 99, 100

thyroid gland, ix, 64, 67, 72, 73

thyroid neoplasms, vii, 43, 45, 52, 54, 55, 65, 66, 67

thyroid nodules, vii, 43, 45, 46, 47, 58, 62, 63, 64, 68, 69

thyroid stimulating hormone, 89

thyroiditis, 44, 47, 49, 54, 60, 64, 67

thyrotropin, 100

tissue, 15, 38, 56, 57, 68, 103, 104, 108, 112, 113, 114, 116, 126

TLR, 4, 14, 34

TLR3, 97

TLR4, 14

TNF, 4, 12, 14

TNF-α, 4, 12

tooth, ix, 123, 125

total cholesterol, 16

total product, 126

toxic effect, viii, 71

toxicity, 14, 72, 73, 80, 85, 86, 89, 90, 94, 106, 107, 127, 132, 133

toxin, 4, 109, 119

TP53, 53, 55, 57, 68, 79

TPA, 4, 14, 26, 39

trade, 9

training, 138

transcription, 4, 12, 14, 17, 20, 22, 26, 29, 30, 35, 36, 37, 38, 41, 51, 60, 74, 80, 83, 85, 86, 94

transcription factors, 12, 30, 94

transcripts, 9, 68, 76

transducer, 4, 80

transformation, 37, 64, 67, 79

transition mutation, 19

translation, 26, 76

translocation, 10, 14, 29, 49, 61

transmission, 137

transplantation, ix, 13, 121, 124, 127

transport, 15, 19, 125

trauma, 125

trial, 19, 23, 35, 38, 70, 80, 87, 88, 91, 92, 99, 100, 107, 110, 111, 114, 115, 116, 121, 129, 132, 144, 146

triangulation, x, 136, 140

triggers, 14, 38, 97

triglycerides, 16

trypsin, 16

tumor cells, viii, 15, 25, 35, 36, 37, 56, 72, 73, 79, 83, 96, 98

tumor development, 77

tumor growth, 12, 14, 15, 20, 26, 34, 40, 52, 79, 83, 85, 94, 97

tumor invasion, 15, 30

tumor necrosis factor, 14, 41
tumor progression, 51, 53, 84
tumorigenesis, 12, 36, 51, 53, 66, 75, 76, 78, 83, 86, 90
tumours, 66, 67
turnover, 127, 128
tyrosine, viii, 4, 12, 21, 37, 48, 49, 54, 61, 67, 72, 75, 76, 78, 83, 84, 87

U

UK, 68
ultrasonography, 47, 62
ultrasound, 45, 62, 63
United Nations, 31
United States (USA), 1, 3, 44, 60, 106, 110
urban, 140
urban areas, 140
urea, 124
urine, 73, 114
urokinase, 26, 39
UV, 77

V

validation, 25, 56, 130
variables, x, 114, 136
variations, 21, 125
vascular accidents, ix, 123
vascular endothelial growth factor (VEGF), 79
vasculature, 15, 25, 85, 119
vector, 121
vegetable oil, 115
vegetables, 5
VEGF expression, 16
VEGFR, 95
viral infection, 128
viscosity, 112, 126
vitamin E, 108
vomiting, 72, 108

W

Washington, 66
water, 84, 102, 103, 111, 114, 124, 128
wear, 115
web, 35, 62
Western blot, 9, 12, 25, 26
Wilcoxon test, x, 136, 140, 141, 142
wild type, 26
Wisconsin, 101
withdrawal, 89
Wnt signaling, 13, 34
workers, 7, 9, 17, 24
World Health Organization (WHO), 4, 5, 8, 19, 31, 44, 54, 136
worldwide, 5, 8, 9, 10, 13, 17, 19, 23, 49, 78
worms, 5
wound healing, 5, 113

X

xanthan gum, 110
xenografts, ix, 12, 20, 33, 40, 72, 80, 83, 84, 85, 93, 98
xerostomia, vii, ix, 101, 102, 103, 104, 105, 106, 107, 108, 109, 110, 111, 112, 113, 114, 115, 116, 117, 118, 119, 120, 121, 123, 125, 126, 127, 128, 129, 130, 131, 132, 133

Y

yeast, 115
yield, viii, 44, 46
young adults, 49

Z

zinc, 20, 128, 132
zinc sulfate, 132